# Wound Management in Urgent Care

Brittany Busse

# Wound Management
# in Urgent Care

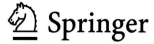 Springer

Brittany Busse, MD
Med 7 Urgent Care
Folsom, CA, USA

ISBN 978-3-319-27426-3      ISBN 978-3-319-27428-7    (eBook)
DOI 10.1007/978-3-319-27428-7

Library of Congress Control Number: 2015958777

Springer Cham Heidelberg New York Dordrecht London

Printed on acid-free paper

Springer International Publishing AG Switzerland is part of Springer Science+Business Media
(www.springer.com)

# Preface

Lacerations, burns, and other wounds are a common reason for patients to present to the Urgent Care. The Center for Disease Control National Center for Health Statistics reports over 3.1 million visits to health care professionals for accidental cutting or piercing injuries in 2012, over 480,000 visits for burns, and over 5.3 million visits for diseases of the skin and subcutaneous tissues (i.e. cellulitis and/or abscess). Many of these patients present to an Urgent Care or Acute Care Center with a variety of acute and chronic wounds. Expedient assessment and treatment is often expected by the patient and leaves little time for the providers to educate themselves on the nuances of surgical wound care.

It is often hard to establish best practice standards in the case of acute and chronic wounds. Lacerations occur in a variety of locations on the body and each wound requires a specialized evaluation and treatment approach. A "one-size fits all" approach to laceration repair can result in suboptimal wound healing and poor patient outcomes. In addition, the treatment of chronic wounds due to illness or neglect on the part of the patient or caregiver can involve a significant level of training and expertise. Due to the difficulty encountered in staying up to date with evidence-based medicine, many providers will fall back on dogma and prior training without realizing that these practices have been shown to lack benefit or may even be harmful to patients.

Complications resulting from inadequate management of wounds early in the course of treatment can include scarring, infection, dehiscence, and/or loss of function of an affected limb. For this reason, many providers may shy away from more complex wounds and instead refer patients to the local Emergency Department, or they may call for the services of a specialist.

The goal of this book is to establish a concise reference to rapidly assist each provider in wound management and increase the provider's overall confidence and competence, which will lead to better patient outcomes.

Folsom, CA, USA                                                                                       Brittany Busse

# Contents

# Chapter 1
# Introduction to Wound Healing

A variety of wound and patient factors affect how and over what period of time a wound heals. Nutritional deficiencies, comorbid diseases, tobacco use, and patient medications can impair wound healing, and this may result in suboptimal outcomes. Also the condition of the wound (whether or not there is devitalized, necrotic, or infected tissue) can impair healing by both primary and secondary intention.

The following chapter addresses the usual time course of wound healing and how it impacts patient care, as well as nutritional advice and treatments to lessen scarring.

## 1.1 Time Course of Wound Healing and Treatment Goals

Wound healing follows a usual pattern whereby cellular components infiltrate the wound and begin the process of breaking down devitalized tissue, preventing infection, and rebuilding collagen. The various stages of wound healing have been well researched and documented over the years [1]. The three stages of wound healing are the result of inflammation, proliferation, and maturation and are delineated by the primary cellular components and soluble factors found in the wound during each time period. The initial stages result in clotting and inflammation, which is followed by migration and proliferation of dermal and epidermal cells to reestablish skin continuity and integrity [2]. Finally these early scars are remodeled to result in mature stable scars with improved elasticity and tensile strength.

Although these stages are distinct, they also overlap [3]. The natural process of wound repair in the body prioritizes filling of the wound followed by reepithelialization and remodeling of the skin and is referred to as healing by secondary intention [4]. When wounds are initially assessed in the urgent care setting, the provider determines whether or not to perform a primary repair of the wound or to allow the wound to heal by secondary intention. The initial steps of a primary repair will facilitate both the filling of the wound gap and restoration of epithelial continuity. The process of wound

© Springer International Publishing Switzerland 2016
B. Busse, *Wound Management in Urgent Care*,
DOI 10.1007/978-3-319-27428-7_1

repair is not significantly altered by this action but it can be sped up dramatically. If done incorrectly, however, a primary repair can result in poorer outcomes than allowing a wound to close by secondary intention. For this reason, adequate assessment is crucial to your role as a medical provider as your actions at the first assessment can affect wound healing efficiency and outcomes.

## 1.1.1  Stage 1 (Days 1–3): Hemostasis and Inflammation

An acute accidental wound or intentional incision will result in loss of epithelial and endothelial integrity. This will initiate the cascade of wound healing starting with hemostasis and inflammation, which are the primary active stages during the first 3 days of wound healing.

Hemostasis and formation of the primary clot are complete within the first minutes to hours (except for patients on anticoagulants or antiplatelet therapy) and are directly followed by the inflammatory phase of wound healing. The key cellular components of this phase of wound healing are platelets, neutrophils, and macrophages.

Platelets are always the first cells to be present in a wound. The role of platelets is to provide immediate primary hemostasis (formation of the blood clot) and to begin the process of creating a new extracellular matrix that will secure the cellular components necessary for wound healing to the wound surface. Many patients may be taking medications such as NSAIDs or Plavix that inhibit the blood clotting function of platelets and make it more difficult to control bleeding. In this case secondary hemostasis may be your first priority when assessing an acute wound.

The secondary function of platelets is to release cytokines, such as platelet-derived growth factor, to attract inflammatory cells to the site of the wound [5]. When exposed collagen fibers in the acute wound interact with platelets, platelet degranulation occurs. Degranulation results in the release of a number of chemotactic factors that will activate the coagulation cascade and lead to the deposition of fibrin in the wound. Fibrin is an integral component of the early wound matrix, and it serves as a scaffold for the migration of later inflammatory cells, the first of which are neutrophils or PMNs.

Inflammatory cells are recruited to the wound site from the wound edges by the chemotactic factors secreted by platelets, the injured endothelial cells, and the clotting factors of the coagulation cascade. PMNs are the first inflammatory cells to arrive in a wound, and their concentration peaks between 24 and 48 h after the initial injury. The primary role of neutrophils is to remove bacteria and debris from the wound by release of enzymes. Although these cells play a vital role in assuring that the tissue is free of any debris and/or infection that would inhibit wound healing, they do not seem to play any role in collagen deposition or wound integrity. Although the inflammatory phase and recruitment of neutrophils is vital to wound closure and repair, chronic inflammation can be detrimental to healing and can lead to loss of wound integrity [6]. As the medical provider assessing an acute wound, it is important to remove any gross contamination of the wound, visibly devitalized or necrotic tissue, and to adequately cleanse, disinfect, and/or irrigate the wound to decrease the bacterial load of the tissue. Gross contamination of the wound can lead to an overly robust inflammatory response that may impair wound healing and continuity.

The second group of inflammatory cells to arrive to the wound is macrophages or activated monocytes. Macrophages are recognized as the most integral cell in wound healing, and their role in inflammation, formation of granulation tissue, and recruitment of other cellular components has been widely researched. The peak concentration of macrophages in the wound is established at around 48 h, and their numbers will fluctuate throughout the inflammatory and proliferation stages, with a continued presence throughout wound healing. Macrophages have phagocytic activity and assist PMNs in removal of debris. They also produce nitric oxide and aid in the antimicrobial activities of neutrophils in the wound. Finally they release cytokines and growth factors that promote collagen deposition and neovascularization. They produce pro-inflammatory cytokines such as tumor necrosis factor alpha, interferon gamma, and interleukins 1, 6, and 12. In most wounds these cells promote recruitment of keratinocytes for reepithelialization, but a prolonged inflammatory phase can lead to poor wound healing, scarring, and fibrosis [7]. Research has shown that macrophage depletion leads to decreased fibroblast recruitment and fibrosis of wounds and that neonatal healing proceeds in the absence of macrophages which may be one of the reasons fetal wounds heal without scaring [8]. However, ongoing research with mice selectively depleted of macrophages prior to injury has shown decreased wound healing, granulation tissue formation, and angiogenesis [9].

The process by which skin integrity is reestablished is called epithelialization, and this process will begin within 1 day of wounding as epidermal cells migrate from wound edges and hair follicles. The formation of granulation tissue is initiated when activated macrophages unite with fibroblasts in the wound bed. These fibroblasts are recruited to the wound by the cytokines produced by activated wound macrophages [7]. Following the formation of granulation tissue, the first stages of reepithelialization occur as keratinocytes migrate inward from the edge of the wounded tissue [6]. The edge of the wound also becomes hyperplastic and thickened as additional epidermal cells begin to proliferate behind the actively migrating fibroblasts, keratinocytes, and epidermal cells [3]. For this reason most wounds that present to the clinic after the first 24 h cannot easily be closed by primary intention as the wounds have already formed a rolled, thickened edge of epidermis that will not seal with direct re-approximation and primary closure.

For normal healthy patients with traumatic wounds closed by primary intention, reepithelialization is typically complete within 48 h. For this reason it is important to carefully instruct patients in the aftercare of re-approximated wounds. In this first 48 h period, it is crucial that patients do not remove or moisten the dressing that was placed while the repaired wound was still sterile. Contaminated water could seep under the edges of the wound during this time and increase the chances of wound infection.

Following the initial 48 h healing period, it is not necessary to apply an antibiotic ointment to a closed wound, and if the patient's daily activities result in minimal trauma to the wound, they may leave it exposed rather than covered with a bandage.

Patients can also wash the area with soap and water and pat it dry gently. This will not affect a wound with appropriate tensile strength, and no bacteria will be able to enter beneath the dermis through a sealed wound.

## 1.1.2   Stage 2: Proliferation

The second stage of wound healing occurs on days 4–12 and is signaled by the appearance of fibroblasts within the wound. At this time granulation tissue begins to proliferate and fill the wounded surface. This granulation tissue is built upon the initial clot or provisional matrix. This provisional matrix is a composite of fibrin, fibronectin, and hyaluronic acid and is used a scaffold for the migration of cellar and vascular components [10]. Macrophages, fibroblasts, and vascular buds are signaled to enter the wound by inflammatory cells of the first phase and they form this initial wound matrix. Macrophages continue to supply growth factors necessary for the recruitment of fibroblasts and angiogenesis [3].

Once localized to the wound, the fibroblasts then begin the process of reestablishing tissue strength and continuity. This is because fibroblasts are the primary ells responsible for collagen synthesis in wounds. Collagen synthesis and cross-linking require an oxygen-rich environment as well as adequate amino acids and cofactors such as vitamin C. After a substantial amount of collagen has been deposited into the wound, the fibroblasts will apoptose and remodeling and vascularization can begin. Abnormal fibroblast function and deregulation of this process leads to fibrotic conditions such as keloid formation and scleroderma [3].

Angiogenesis is initiated starting with tissue injury and hypoxemia, followed by release of growth factors from migrating cells. Activated epidermal cells in the wound secrete large amounts of vascular endothelial growth factors [3]. Endothelial cells also proliferate during this phase of wound healing leading to neovascularization or the formation of new blood vessels within the wound. New capillary tubule formation is often exaggerated during this phase of wound healing leading to the characteristic reddish/pink color of newly formed scars.

## 1.1.3   Stage 3: Scar Maturation and Remodeling

The final stage of wound healing is maturation and remodeling of collagen. At this time the wound begins to achieve increased tensile strength through collagen cross-linking and the morphological change of fibroblasts into myofibroblasts. At about 10 days following the acute injury, collagen synthesis and wound tensile strength have increased dramatically, but are still only about 20 % of normal skin. Collagen is continuously degraded and synthesized during this period into an arrangement of greater stability. Tensile strength is the greatest contributor to healing wounds by primary intention, which is what most providers will be faced with in the urgent care setting. For this reason, patients with favorable wounds and no comorbid diseases and who are relatively young can have the sutures or staples removed from their wounds at day 10 or sooner for wounds without tension (this will be discussed later in the book). Scarred tissue will never regain full strength and maximum tensile strength will be about 70–80 % of unwounded tissues.

Patients will be concerned with the appearance of the scar and how to lessen scarring. There is no evidence at this time to support the use of any over-the-counter or homeopathic treatment as there has been little to no subjective improvement in scar appearance with their use and the trials so far conducted have been of poor quality [11]. Minimal cost interventions that have been shown to have a small benefit, and are of little to no harm, would be application of *Aloe vera* gel or vitamin E oil.

**Instructions for Aftercare**
- The initial closure should be kept clean, dry, and covered for 48 h with a sterile to semi-sterile dressing.
- After 48 h the skin is sealed. Do not apply topical antimicrobials (moisture will weaken the integrity of the healing wound). Patients can choose to keep the sutures covered or open depending on the location.
- No soaking of wounds in water, but showering, as well as handwashing with soap, and then lightly patting dry, is okay.
- Patients with wounds on the upper extremity including shoulder girdle should be kept from lifting over 10 lb for the first 10–14 days.

# Chapter 2
# Improving Outcomes in Wound Healing

Wound healing can be impaired by a variety of wound-specific factors including the presence of bacteria, debris, and/or devitalized tissue. Other factors which affect wound healing are patient conditions that can result in decreased function of immune cells and poor oxygenation of tissues, such as smoking, diabetes, peripheral vascular disease, poor nutritional status, steroid, and immune-modulating or cytotoxic drugs. These and other factors can contribute to poor blood flow and wound ischemia, resulting in poorly healing wounds and dehiscence.

## 2.1  Local Wound Environment

In the primary assessment and prior to wound closure, you must establish that the wound is free of excessive contamination or devitalized tissue. The reason for this is simple; devitalized tissue, foreign bodies, and excessive contamination will increase the chances of wound infection. Wound infection can lead to increased inflammation, scarring, wound dehiscence, prolonged healing, severe cellulitis, and decreased functionality. Wound irrigation is the most important aspect of wound preparation as it is the primary way that excessive contamination is removed from acute traumatic wounds [12]. The process of adequate irrigation and debridement will be covered again later in the text. Multiple studies have attempted to determine the optimal method and amount of irrigation needed to significantly reduce bacterial load and risk of infection. So far there has been a clear benefit demonstrated in irrigation versus no irrigation, but no specific method has been shown to have a statistically significant benefit over any other method [12]. For this reason, I recommend a simple syringe-based method for pressurized irrigation of the wound. Prior to infiltration of anesthetic, cleanse the wound edges using chlorhexidine gluconate (Hibiclens) or povidone-iodine diluted in water or normal saline. Take care not to get these agents in the wound as they can cause pain and disruption of the cellular components necessary for wound healing. After the wound has been anesthetized, irrigate

© Springer International Publishing Switzerland 2016
B. Busse, *Wound Management in Urgent Care*,
DOI 10.1007/978-3-319-27428-7_2

the wound with normal saline solution. Pressure irrigation can be performed using a syringe and a splatter shield. Depending on the size of the wound, 100–200 cm³ of fluid should be utilized for adequate irrigation. At this point foreign material still remaining in the wound can be removed with a forceps, and devitalized tissue can be removed using a forceps and tissue scissors.

**Cleansing Around a Wound**
- Hibiclens or iodine (do not use Hibiclens near the mouth or eyes).
- Cleanse three times with a new sterile gauze or swab soaked in the antimicrobial agent of choice.
- Cleanse from the wound in a circle extending outward.

Time of presentation of the acute wound was at one time felt to influence the local wound environment. Wounds >6–8 h old were often left open due to the fact that it was believed they represented a higher infection risk. Current research has shown this to be a false assumption [13]. Wounds can be successfully closed at less than 24 h without any additional intervention, aside from irrigation. After this point wound epithelialization may have an impact on wound closure but not infection.


## 2.2  Infection

Wound infections can lead to morbidity of wounds including wound dehiscence, disfiguring scarring, and delayed closures. Identifying and treating infections early can lead to improved wound closure outcomes.

During the initial treatment of the acute traumatic wound, application of a topical antimicrobial after wound closure has been shown to effectively reduce the rate of infection. The compounds most effective at preventing infection, while also minimizing associated complications, were found to be bacitracin zinc and neomycin sulfate [14].

Patients should be carefully instructed so that they know how to examine the wound daily for increasing redness, pain, swelling, or discharge from the wound site that might indicate the presence of infection. They should have the ability to return for evaluation as needed during the period between wound closure and suture removal. Patients should typically be seen 2 days after wound closure and treatment for removal of the initial dressing and assessment for wound infection. If wound infection is suspected, one or two sutures or staples should be removed, and a sterile cotton swab can be used to open the wound to probe for purulence. If purulence is expressed, the wound should be opened adequately and thoroughly irrigated to allow drainage of the infection. Antibiotics should only be given when there is extensive cellulitis of the tissues surrounding the wound (>1 cm surrounding erythema or lymphangitis).

There is no benefit to prophylactic antibiotic usage in acute wounds, and this may lead to the emergence of antibiotic-resistant organisms. In addition wounds should be carefully assessed for pathologic versus physiologic inflammation. Many healing wounds will present with a peripheral erythema of about 2–5 mm surrounding the wound. This is not an indication of infection but simply a normal wound healing process. Prudent use of antibiotics should also be tailored to the organisms most likely to be infecting the wound. For the majority of patients, a first-generation cephalosporin (or clindamycin for patients with an allergy to cephalosporins) with activity against *Staphylococcus aureus* and *Streptococcus* sp. (such as cephalexin) is adequate. Unless the patient has known history of methicillin-resistant *Staphylococcus aureus* (MRSA) or other risk factors (multiple hospitalizations, multiple infections, IV drug use, etc.), it is not necessary to use a broad-spectrum antibiotic such as TMP-sulfa, doxycycline, or levofloxacin. The overuse of these drugs is leading to the emergence of new resistance patterns in *Staphylococcus* and *Streptococcus* species.

## 2.3  Age

Although systemic factors may not always be under the direct control of the provider or of the patient, efforts should be made to correct any modifiable risk factors. Age, for instance, is not a modifiable risk factor, but it should be taken into account when determining when to remove sutures from an elderly population. Advanced age leads to alterations in inflammation and cellular interactions that can prolong and impair epithelial and endothelial cell binding and interactions. This can lead to an increase in the risk of wound dehiscence in elderly patients. In a study conducted on otherwise healthy human volunteers, it was determined that patients over the age of 70 required an additional 1.9 days of healing compared to a younger population of patients [15].

In addition, many elderly patients may suffer from comorbid conditions that negatively affect wound healing such as cardiovascular disease, diabetes, nutritional deficiencies, and autoimmune diseases and may take a variety of medications that may or may not be known to impair wound healing and collagen integrity such as immune-modulating agents and corticosteroids. For this reason it may be prudent to allow 2–4 additional days for wound healing or to apply adhesive strips for added wound support following the removal sutures from acute wounds in elderly patients.

## 2.4  Local Tissue Hypoxemia

Poor oxygenation of tissue can have a deleterious effect on wound healing. Poor oxygenation impairs the function of neutrophils and can result in increased infection and dehiscence rates of wounds [16]. The number one modifiable risk factor to improve oxygenation in wound healing is cessation of tobacco use.

Collagen synthesis requires oxygen as a cofactor and local tissue hypoxemia can lead to loss of epithelial integrity. Nicotine is a highly vasoconstrictive compound that has been shown to prolong the healing time of wounds in otherwise healthy indviduals [17]. Tissue hypoxemia from blood vessel constriction due to tobacco use can also impair the function of fibroblasts, thereby decreasing collagen synthesis and cross-linking. Patients who smoke also tend to suffer from higher rates of wound complications such as infection and dehiscence due to impaired cellular mechanisms and collagen cross-linking as described.

Other factors that can lead to decreased tissue oxygenation are tissue edema and excessive tension on the wounds. For wounds on edematous extremities, patients should be counseled on compression and elevation of affected extremities, and efforts should be made to control underlying diseases such as heart failure. Excessive tension is under the direct control of the provider. Oftentimes direct tension on the wound can be alleviated by disruption of the subcutaneous fibrous connections between the dermis and the subdermal components.

## 2.5  Diabetes

Uncontrolled diabetes has a number of detrimental effects on wound healing, and diabetic patients should understand the added importance of good glucose control during the healing period. It is the number one metabolic disorder that affects wound healing as it has detrimental effects on oxygenation, growth factor signaling, neovascularization, and immune function [18]. Poorly controlled diabetes decreases the number and availability of small blood vessels contributing to tissue hypoxemia. In addition glycosylation of proteins decreases the overall amount of growth factors and signaling proteins available during the inflammatory phase of wound healing. Impaired glucose utilization also negatively impacts neutrophils and fibroblasts leading to increased risk of infections and decreased collagen synthesis.

## 2.6  Nutrition

The importance of nutrition as a modifiable risk factor should not be overlooked, especially in elderly, frail, or chronically ill patients, some of which may present to an urgent care with an acute or chronic wound for evaluation [19]. Patients may also inquire of you how to improve their own outcomes both in terms of wound integrity and decreased scarring. It is important to counsel patients that adequate protein intake has been correlated with improved outcomes in wound healing and repair, although increase in the amount of protein ingested does not correlate with improved healing. Ensuring that patients are not significantly malnourished at the time of presentation (especially in the elderly and those completely dependent upon others for care) is more important than advising patients to take in an excess of protein.

In addition, vitamins A and C are necessary cofactors for wound healing and collagen synthesis. Deficiencies in protein, vitamin A, and vitamin C have been linked with increased rates of infection as well as poor wound healing and dehiscence. Vitamin C supplementation, however, has not been shown to improve wound healing. This is likely because vitamin C is a water-soluble vitamin, and excess amounts will be lost in urine. Vitamin A supplementation of 25,000 to 100,000 IU have been advocated to improve wound healing, decrease infection by increasing the effectiveness of the inflammatory phase of wound healing, and increasing collagen synthesis and epidermal cell replication and growth even in non-deficient healthy populations [20]. Vitamin A has also been shown to improve impaired wound healing in patients currently taking steroids [21] or those who have diabetes and other chronic illnesses.

Another trace element that has been studied extensively in wound healing is zinc. Zinc is a critical cofactor for a number of enzymes that are integral to wound healing [22]. Many critical aspects of wound healing are impaired in zinc-deficient patients, but at this time there has been no clear benefit shown to zinc supplementation in normal, non-deficient patient populations.

# Chapter 3
# Treatment of Acute Wounds: The Basics

There are certain steps you should follow each and every time you assess an acute wound to ensure proper management and optimal outcome for the patient. Having an established algorithm by which you evaluate and treat patients will improve consistency and decrease morbidity.

1. Begin with a thorough evaluation of the wound type and depth.
2. After you have determined it is appropriate to treat the wound in the urgent care clinic, prepare for wound closure.
3. Finally close the wound using appropriate materials.

The next chapter will go over each of these steps in detail to assist you in providing optimal treatment for each and every wound.

## 3.1  Evaluation

When the patient presents to the clinic with an acute wound, you will need to quickly assess the wound as well as the patient.

The patient should have a brief but thorough history focusing on factors that may complicate wound closure and healing including medications that may inhibit hemostasis (aspirin, Plavix, or Coumadin), history of bleeding or clotting disorders, concomitant illnesses, use of immunomodulatory medications and/or corticosteroids, tobacco use, and date of last tetanus vaccination. Patients who have not had tetanus toxoid vaccination in the past 5 years should be offered the immunization at the time of intervention. If the patient appears unstable (tachycardia, diaphoresis, pallor, or hypotension), attempt to control bleeding and call 911 for immediate transport.

The wound should be assessed for depth and damage to underlying structures. Wounds to the thorax or abdomen with injury to the muscle fascia should have

© Springer International Publishing Switzerland 2016
B. Busse, *Wound Management in Urgent Care*,
DOI 10.1007/978-3-319-27428-7_3

immediate transport to a trauma center by calling 911. To avoid missing a potential tendon injury, passive and active range of motion of the extremity should be examined. Performing the examination while inspecting the inside of the wound is optimal so you can assess for any fraying of the tendon. More proximal wounds should be evaluated for damage to the muscle body that may impair functionality of the limb. Next evaluate for injuries to nerves by carefully assessing distal innervation. There may be slight numbness distal to the wound, however; two-point discrimination should be intact. When the wound may involve a joint capsule, it is important that you have the capability to perform a saline arthrogram. If this is not in your scope of practice, the patient should be referred elsewhere. If there is any possibility of tendon damage, joint involvement, muscle involvement, or an open fracture, you should not attempt to close the wound in the urgent care clinic. Each of these situations would require specialized assessment and intervention by a specialist for optimal results.

Examination of the wound should also include an assessment for nonviable tissue as well as foreign bodies that could complicate wound healing or cause infection. As discussed earlier, most of the foreign material and contamination will be removed during irrigation, but for penetrating wounds with small openings, this may not adequately rule out retained foreign bodies. If you have the capabilities, it would be important to obtain an X-ray prior to closure of the wound to ensure there are no radiopaque foreign bodies deep within the wound. The patient history providing mechanism of injury will help you to determine how thorough the evaluation for foreign bodies in the wound needs to be.

## 3.2   Prepare the Wound

Preparation of the wound for closure has five parts: hemostasis, cleansing, anesthesia, debridement, and irrigation.

### 3.2.1   Hemostasis

Hemostasis may be achieved by holding direct pressure (with one or two fingers depending on the size of the wound) or, in the case of extremities, by placing a temporary occlusive device proximally such as a tourniquet. A finger tourniquet can be quickly fashioned by cutting the long finger of a rubber glove and tying it securely around the finger proximal to the wound. If you find it necessary to apply a tourniquet, remember to work quickly as the tissue distal to the tourniquet is being deprived of oxygen. This will increase the risk of wound complications like infection and dehiscence. Avoid placing tourniquets proximally on extremities in the urgent care, unless you are planning to transfer the patient to a higher level of care.

### 3.2.2 Cleansing

The skin around the wound should be cleansed with an antimicrobial solution of either dilute chlorhexidine gluconate or providone-iodine. This will decrease the amount of skin flora around the wound prior to closure and also decrease the chances of inoculating bacteria into the soft tissues during the injection of anesthetic. As discussed previously, take care not to get these solutions in the wound itself. Antimicrobial solutions inhibit cellular activity resulting in poor wound healing. After you have cleansed the skin surrounding the wound, place a sterile field around the wound. This is to prevent contamination of suture material and other equipment during wound repair.

### 3.2.3 Anesthesia

Once you have achieved hemostasis, you should anesthetize the wound. Lidocaine (1 or 2 %) with or without epinephrine (1:100,000 dilution) is the preferred method of local anesthesia for acute wound care. Epinephrine should be deferred in wounds of the fingers, toes, ears, nose, and penis as the infiltration of epinephrine can theoretically cause spasm of the small arterioles resulting in tissue necrosis and impaired wound healing. Local anesthetic infiltration can cause significant patient discomfort. It is important to discuss this with the patient before you begin so that the patient is aware. Because small children may not fully comprehend that the pain of infiltration will be limited and will prevent pain later on in the procedure, I find it helpful to explain it to them in detail and with very finite terms. I have the children count to 10 or 20 (whatever amount of time you think you need to adequately infiltrate the wound) and tell them that when they get to 10 or 20, the pain will be over and there will be no other pain during the procedure. Also the addition of a buffer of sodium bicarbonate can reduce the burning sensation that accompanies local injection, although it does not eliminate it completely. For every 5 cm$^3$ of lidocaine, I recommend 1 cm$^3$ of sodium bicarbonate. Performing a digital block for local anesthesia will be discussed in more detail in the chapter on finger/toe lacerations.

### 3.2.4 Debridement

After you have obtained adequate anesthesia of the wound, you should perform a more thorough evaluation of the depth of the wound. At this time you should remove any foreign bodies from the wound and debride the wound of any nonviable tissue. At this time you should remove any blood clots that have formed in the wound and search for bleeding vessels. These vessels can be cauterized if necessary or ligated with a suture. Do not suture ligate bleeding vessels in the fingers. The remaining suture has a very high likelihood to act as a nidus for infection and this should be avoided at all costs. Also the distal circulation of the finger is completely dependent on two sets of vessels. If one is ligated, it will impair circulation to the finger and cause significant tissue damage. If any of the wound edges appear congested (purplish) or necrotic (black), these should be trimmed back to viable tissue before re-approximation, as they will only impair wound closure. Don't overly debride the wounds though, as you will want to have enough tissue remaining for wound closure without undue tension.

## 3.2.5   Irrigation

You should then irrigate the wound with normal saline without any additives to remove debris and bacterial contamination. As stated previously, there is no agreed upon way to pressure irrigate an acute wound, but irrigation with a syringe and splatter shield provides enough pressure to significantly decrease the risk of infection compared to no irrigation. Be sure to use at least 100–200 mL of sterile saline. Do not cleanse inside of wounds with iodine or hydrogen peroxide as this has been shown to impair wound healing by damaging the macrophages and neutrophils within the wound.

## 3.3   Wound Closure

Now that you have evaluated and prepared the wound, it is time for the closure. Specific suture types and closure techniques for wounds in different anatomical locations will be addressed in the chapters to follow.

## 3.3.1   Layered Closure

Approximation of the deep layers of wounds should be undertaken only if the wound includes a layer of fascia. This may be the muscle fascia or a subcutaneous fascia as is found in wounds of the face, arms, legs, and trunk.

### Sterile Gloves
Sterile gloves should be utilized during wound repair. A pair of non-latex, powder-free gloves are optimal as many patients may suffer from latex allergy and powder has been shown to increase the rate of infection and inflammatory fibrosis in wounds.

Deep sutures should never be placed into fat. This tissue has very poor blood supply and tensile strength. It will not hold the sutures and will pull apart resulting in fat necrosis in the wound. This suture material and necrotic fat can lead to inflammation and infection within the wound.

Do not attempt to place deep sutures into hands, feet, fingers, or toes. They have no subcutaneous fascial layers.

Multilayer closures should be used sparingly as they are associated with a higher risk of infection. Additional foreign body within the wound can become a nidus for infection and should only be used when there is a definite indication (i.e., wound spreading due to involvement of the fascia or for closure of wounds without undue tension.)

Deep layers should be closed with braided, absorbable suture of the smallest caliber necessary to hold the wound without tension, typically 4-0 or 5-0 Vicryl or equivalent.

### 3.3.2   Superficial Closure

Once the deep tissues have been approximated and the wound is no longer under tension, you can close the superficial wound. The skin edges should be carefully re-approximated with staples or nonabsorbable sutures. Clinical reasoning for selection of particular material will be presented in the following chapters. Precise re-approximation by bisection is the best way to achieve optimal cosmesis. In wounds with cornered edges, corners should be re-approximated first. Special precision needs to be taken with re-approximation of eyebrows, the hairline, and the vermillion border of the lip. If the wound is not precisely re-approximated in these areas, the results will be immediately obvious to patients. If you do not feel comfortable with approximating certain wounds, then the patient should be referred to a local hospital, potentially one with plastic surgical capabilities if available.

# Chapter 4
# Selecting Materials for Wound Closure

You should have several basic kinds of suture available to you for wound closure including monofilament nonabsorbable, monofilament absorbable, and braided absorbable material. The following chapter will go through the different types of sutures, where they are best utilized, the sizing system, and the type and size of the needle. This chapter also addresses when to use staples, liquid tissue adhesives, or adhesive strips.

## 4.1 Monofilament Nonabsorbable Suture

When repairing wounds and laceration caused by accidental trauma, you will likely select a monofilament nonabsorbable suture for an interrupted closure. The reason for this is to minimize the chance for infection. Absorbable monofilament and braided multifilament absorbable sutures are more likely to harbor microbes beneath the surface of the skin, thus increasing the risk of an infection in a contaminated wound.

The go-to nonabsorbable monofilament suture for superficial laceration repair is typically a synthetic material such as nylon (Ethilon/Monosof) or polypropylene (Prolene). All foreign bodies including suture cause localized tissue reaction but this seems to be less for synthetics like nylon and polypropylene versus silk [23]. One major drawback of silk suture use on the skin is the robust initial inflammatory reaction, which can lead to fibrosis and increased collagen deposition. This can result in fibrotic and cosmetically inferior scarring, so the recommendation would be to use a good multipurpose suture like nylon or polypropylene for all skin-level repair of lacerations and acute wounds.

Synthetic suture also has greater tensile strength as compared to silk suture [23]. They are more pliable and easier to handle for knot tie-down than natural monofilament sutures. One drawback can be that they tend to hold memory, which is the folding of

© Springer International Publishing Switzerland 2016
B. Busse, *Wound Management in Urgent Care*,
DOI 10.1007/978-3-319-27428-7_4

the suture within the package, and need to be held to tension prior to use to release the memory out of the material.

Synthetic materials also cause less tissue drag and sheering and are utilized predominantly in cosmetic surgery and on delicate tissues.

One role for silk suture that can be addressed here is its utility for tying off bleeding vessels. Silk suture is the material preferred by surgeons for hemostasis, as well as for internal anastomoses, as it is actually dissolved by proteolysis and removed from the body within 2 years unlike synthetic materials such as nylon and polypropylene which are hydrolyzed slowly but retained in the tissues due to encapsulation over prolonged periods of time. As mentioned previously in the section on hemostasis, suture ligation should never be attempted in the digits, but may be helpful to control bleeding of large-caliber vessels in more proximal wounds.

## 4.2   Monofilament Absorbable Suture

Natural monofilament absorbable sutures come in three types but are all derived from the same process. These collagen-based sutures derived from the submucosa of the ovine small intestine are referred to as "gut" sutures. Gut sutures are available in 3 types: plain, fast absorbing, and chromic. Plain gut is rarely used in acute wound care but fast-absorbing and chromic gut sutures have utility in two very specific circumstances.

Fast-absorbing gut suture maintains its tensile strength and stability for 5–7 days and can be used for epidermal closure of acute lacerations on the faces of children. The advantage of this material for this purpose is that it will rapidly break down and is easily removed without cutting, thus sparing the child the added distress of suture removal.

Chromic gut is coated with chromium salts, which helps to delay enzymatic degradation. This type of suture material is ideal for use inside the mouth on the mucosal surfaces, as it will maintain its integrity for about 7–14 days while the tissue heals itself [24].

One drawback of natural filament absorbable suture is that it is delicate and can fray easily, which means that knot tie-down can be more difficult than with nonabsorbable suture. It can also cause tissue damage due to friction and should be pulled through delicate tissues carefully. I recommend using it only for the above two indications and if you are familiar with its handling.

Other types of absorbable monofilament sutures are typically not utilized in acute wound care. Materials such as poliglecaparone-25 (Monocryl) are reserved for running subcuticular closures in sterile surgical procedures. This material could potentially harbor microbes below the surface of accidental and contaminated acute wounds and would need to be removed in its entirety in the case of infection. Whereas if you use nonabsorbable monofilaments in an epidermal interrupted closure, then just one or two sutures can be removed to allow purulence to drain from an infected wound. The difference in healing between nonabsorbable and absorbable sutures has been studied in traumatic wounds. No significant difference was noted in the healing of the wounds or cosmetic outcome; however, the absorbable suture has been shown to have a higher number of complication [25].

## 4.3 Braided (Multifilament) Absorbable Suture

Polyglactin-910 (Vicryl) suture is a multipurpose multifilament absorbable suture that is the only one you will need in your laceration repair arsenal. Its strengths include ease of use, ease of knot tie-down, high tensile strength, and prolonged absorption. It causes very little tissue inflammation and fibrosis, but one major drawback is suture extrusion when used in subcuticular suturing. The major use of Vicryl will be for layered closure in acute wounds that extend through the subdermal fascia of the extremities and torso. Multifilament sutures should only be used to close deep fascial layers with natural collagenous tensile strength. They should never be placed in fat or below the surface of the epidermis in the feet, toes, hands, or fingers. Multifilament sutures can cause fat necrosis when inappropriately placed in fat without subcutaneous fascia, which can increase the risk of infection.

## 4.4 Needle Selection

There are a wide variety of needle types and sizes in today's commercially available sutures. Selecting one type that will work well in multiple situations will be most economical in the urgent or acute care setting. Ideally you will select a small needle with appropriate curvature that will be stable in a needle holder. A needle with a three-eighths inch curvature has been shown to be optimal for skin closure. The needle length is provided on the package. Typically a 13 mm needle length is ideal for skin closure in all situations no matter the size of the suture (4-0, 5-0, or 6-0). Finally, you will select the needle type (blunt, cutting, or reverse cutting). A reverse cutting needle has the cutting edge on the outside (convex side) of the needle and is optimal for causing minimal trauma to the skin [26]. Conventional cutting needles with the cutting edge on the inside (concave side) of the needle cause increased tissue damage and are typically reserved for denser tissues.

For absorbable suture that will be used in approximation of the fascia, it is recommended to have a taper or round-point needle that will gently spread the tissue. This is because this tissue is typically easily penetrated but will tear if cut too deeply.

## 4.5 Selecting an Appropriately Sized Suture

The optimal suture is always the smallest size that provides appropriate tensile strength for the wound you are closing. I recommend going no larger than a 4-0 suture for all types of acute wounds. For those requiring increased tensile strength,

I would recommend familiarizing yourself with the horizontal and vertical mattress interrupted suturing technique that will be presented in a later chapter.

Regions of the face and neck require suture with very little tensile strength and will be most scrutinized by patients for scarring. For this reason selecting a very small (6-0) monofilament nonabsorbable suture with low drag such as polypropylene or nylon will optimize the cosmetic result.

Other regions under slightly more tension include the dorsal surface of the hands, arms, and feet, as well as the upper chest, and should be closed with a slightly larger nonabsorbable suture (5-0). Arguably the volar forearm, other than the flexion surface of the wrist, is also under very little tension compared to other areas and could be closed with 5-0 suture as well.

All other surfaces will require 4-0 nonabsorbable suture to provide the appropriate tensile strength during movement. It is inappropriate to splint sutured regions for prolonged periods of time. Appropriately selected suture size and correct knot tie-down will prevent sheering of tissues and unraveling of suture during the healing process.

## 4.6  Stainless Steel Staples

Stainless steel staple provide excellent approximation of wounds under tension and in those areas where scarring will be less noticeable such as regions covered by hair. I recommend using staples for wound closure over joints (knee, elbow), on the scalp, and on the lower leg. If removed in 7–10 days, they are no more likely to cause inflammation or "railroad track" markings than suture, and they provide optimal closure against tension, thus preventing most cases of wound dehiscence and prolonged healing by secondary intention.

## 4.7  Wound Closure with Adhesive Strips

Wound closure tapes should be reserved only for very small wounds (less than 1–2 cm) that occur in areas with very little tension such as the face and tips of the fingers. Another important caveat is that the wound should already be hemostatic as bleeding can interfere with placement of the tape. Benzoin should be applied to the wound edges to sterilize them and to add additional tackiness to the closure. Wounds should be closed from the side of greater tension to the more stable side. Tapes should not be used on skin tears as they can cause additional trauma with removal. Numerous studies of the use of adhesive tape in wound closure have shown no significant difference in cosmesis compared to suturing.

Finally, adhesive strip application after suture removal can provide support to healing wounds in anatomical locations under tension or in the elderly.

## 4.8   Octyl Cyanoacrylate Tissue Adhesive

The use of the liquid tissue adhesive is very similar to that of adhesive strips but can provide increased support to healing tissues with superior burst strength than wound closure tapes. Use of tissue glue has not been shown to increase the rates of infection when used in contaminated wounds and has been shown to provide superior cosmetic results in small, simple, linear wounds with viable edges [27]. The application of tissue glue is also preferred in small children with appropriate wound characteristics, as its use will cause significantly less emotional trauma. Finally tissue glue is the preferred method of closure of skin tears in the elderly, which will be addressed in a later chapter.

# Chapter 5
# Proper Setup

Before you start there are a few more points on setup of which you should be aware.

## 5.1 Surgical Tray Setup

The contents of your surgical tray should include necessary instruments for wound repair. You should have a small sterile basin for sterile saline and chlorhexidine or iodine for wound cleansing as well as a reasonable amount of sterile gauze. A surgical tray should contain an 18G needle for drawing up anesthetic as well as a 25G needle for anesthetizing the skin. The surgical instruments should include a smooth edge needle driver of appropriate size and length (typically 12 cm). A smooth edge to the jaws is optimal for smaller-caliber (5-0 and 6-0) sutures and will be adequate for any 4-0 Vicryl that may be used for deep suturing. The smooth edge prevents breakage of the finer monofilament strands, which can occur with textured jaw needle drivers. In addition pickups (forceps/tweezers) with teeth are preferable to one with smooth edges. The reason for this is that the teeth can be used to gently grasp rather than crush the edges of the tissue. Apply only the smallest amount of pressure necessary to grasp the tissue edge rather than crushing it between the jaws of the pickups. You are not using the forceps to grasp the needle; this is the role of the needle driver. Finally two pairs of scissors should be included in the tray, a small sharp scissors for debridement of devitalized tissue and a larger scissors for cutting suture. The reason for this is twofold. The smaller pair should be kept very sharp to prevent crushing of healthy tissue during debridement. Cutting of the suture material can dull the edge of the scissors after multiple cuts and so a separate scissor should be kept on hand for cutting of suture.

© Springer International Publishing Switzerland 2016
B. Busse, *Wound Management in Urgent Care*,
DOI 10.1007/978-3-319-27428-7_5

## 5.2   Positioning of the Needle

This may seem like a small point but proper positioning of the needle in the needle driver will allow you to more easily enter the skin at a 90° angle causing minimal trauma to the tissue and setting you up for a proper wound closure. Appropriate needle and needle holder interaction will result in greater precision and control during wound repair.

The needle holder should be of appropriate size for the needle that you are using. A needle holder that is too large will cause the needle to straighten due to uneven pressure, while a needle holder that is too small will cause the needle to be unstable within the needle holder.

The needle should be grasped slightly off-center, nearer the swage end (the end attached to the suture) than the needle tip. The needle should be held within the needle holder with a slight cant away from the operator to allow for easier insertion into the tissue when the hand is pronated. Thus the needle and suture can be brought smoothly through the tissue when the hand is supinated. This results in greater precision as well as great comfort to the medical practitioner performing the wound repair.

# Chapter 6
# Suturing Techniques for Wound Closure

There are three different suturing techniques that you should be familiar with for the closure of traumatic wounds. These are simple interrupted closure, horizontal mattress technique, and vertical mattress technique.

## 6.1 Simple Interrupted Closure

This is the most commonly used technique for repair of acute wounds. The needle should enter the skin about 1–2 mm from the edge at a 90° angle with the hand in slight over-pronation. The hand is then supinated to bring the curve of the needle through the skin and out through the wound. The needle is then repositioned in the needle driver. This time the needle enters just below the dermis as the hand is supinated, and the needle emerges from the skin about 1–2 mm from the wound edge. The two ends of the suture can then be brought together and securely tied without undue pressure or tension on the skin.

## 6.2 Horizontal Mattress Suture Technique

The horizontal mattress suture technique should be utilized for wounds requiring eversion to decrease tension over the wound's length. Examples would be wounds of convex surfaces such as the arm, torso, and upper leg. This type of wound closure can also be used for fragile skin including those in patients with impaired wound healing capabilities due to comorbid illness.

The horizontal mattress suture should enter the skin perpendicularly with the hand slightly over-pronated, like the simple interrupted suture, except it should enter

© Springer International Publishing Switzerland 2016
B. Busse, *Wound Management in Urgent Care*,
DOI 10.1007/978-3-319-27428-7_6

about 4–5 mm from the wound edge exiting about 4–5 mm from the opposite edge (after repositioning of the needle in the center as described above for simple interrupted suture placement). At this point the needle is placed backward into the needle driver, and the skin is entered about 5 mm distally coming back across the wound and exiting again on the proximal side. At this point the two ends of the suture can be tied off being very careful not to put too much tension or pressure on the skin, but just enough to slightly evert the wound edges. It is very important to enter and exit at the same distance on both sides to prevent step-offs on the wound and uneven/thickened scarring. This method of repair can also result in tissue necrosis if undue pressure is placed on the skin. Be sure to tie off the ends gently, placing just enough tension to lightly approximate and evert the edges.

## 6.3  Vertical Mattress Suture Technique

The vertical mattress suture technique can also be employed to evert the skin edges, but is less commonly used than the horizontal mattress suture technique. This technique can provide eversion without tension in regions of the body with a very thick epidermis, such as on the posterior neck and back.

The vertical mattress suture is typically placed using the far-far, near-near technique. The skin is entered about 4–5 mm from the wound edge proximally and exits about 4–5 mm from the wound edge distally. This initial suture should cross deep to the dermis. The needle is then placed backward in the needle driver and brought from distal to proximal starting approximately 1–2 mm from the wound edge and coming out through the mid-epidermis, then entering at the same level and exiting 1–2 mm from the edge on the proximal side. The two ends of the suture are then carefully tied off without undue pressure or tension and carefully everting the wound edge to prevent step-offs as with the horizontal mattress technique.

# Chapter 7
# Specifics of Wound Closure

The following section will break down wound closure for specific anatomical regions of the body and will be most useful as a quick reference guide for wound closure in the acute setting.

## 7.1 Scalp

Before embarking on evaluation and repair of scalp lacerations, first evaluate the patient. Scalp lacerations can be the cause of significant hemorrhage, even before the patient arrives to the urgent care. If the patient is pale, hypotensive, clammy, or tachycardic, or if they have signs of intracranial injury such as loss of consciousness, nausea, vomiting, headache, dizziness, or unequal/unresponsive pupils, call 911 for immediate transport to the Emergency Department.

When evaluating the wound, it is important to note that there are five layers of the scalp, but only the first three are important to acute wound care in the urgent care setting. The first layer is the epidermis, which is covered with dense hair. Ragged edges of epidermis should be debrided as at some point this scar may become visible (short haircuts, balding, etc.). The second layer is the superficial fascia, which is a dense layer of connective tissue containing a vast network of arteries and veins. This layer of connective tissue is what tends to hold scalp wounds open and causes profuse early bleeding from even small lacerations. There is no need to perform deep closure of this layer as it will be brought together adequately by standard wound closure with stainless steel staples (preferred) or 4-0 monofilament (nylon or prolene) suture. The final layer to be concerned about is the galea aponeurotica or the tendinous layer of the muscles of the face and scalp. If there is a large laceration to the frontalis portion of the galea, it must be

© Springer International Publishing Switzerland 2016

B. Busse, *Wound Management in Urgent Care*,

DOI 10.1007/978-3-319-27428-7_7

repaired. If left open the frontalis muscle may contract unevenly causing cosmetic deformity of the brow. It would be very rare to encounter a laceration through the galea in the urgent care and if found on evaluation may prompt you to send the patient to the Emergency Department.

There are several alternatives for obtaining closure of a scalp laceration: suturing, staples, or hair apposition. Advantages of suturing are security of wound closure and adequate eversion of skin edges leading to improved cosmesis, and it is preferred for wounds requiring layered closure [28]. Disadvantages of suture include the need for adequate infiltration of anesthetic, which can cause increased bleeding and poor visualization of scalp wounds, as well as increased patient discomfort. Studies have also shown increased complications with suturing including redness, scarring, hair loss, and infection [29]. In my experience, stainless steel staples are the preferred method for wound closure of the scalp. Advantages include less patient discomfort (topical lidocaine-epinephrine can easily be used as an anesthetic because the staples penetrate with less depth than sutures), more expedient than suturing, and less risk of injury to the care provider [30]. This is especially important in a pediatric population. The final method discussed for closure of scalp laceration is referred to as hair apposition technique and was initially described by Hock et al. in 2002 [31]. The method involves taking 4–5 strands of hair from each side of the wound, crossing them, and then securing them with tissue glue. This is done at regular intervals until the wound is closed. Retrospective and randomized controlled studies of this technique have shown advantages of improved patient satisfaction, decreased pain, and improved cosmesis (decreased scarring compared to suturing) [32].

Hair removal is not necessary prior to sutured or stapled closure of scalp wounds as hair contains only small amounts of bacteria that are easily removed with standard wound cleansing.

Scalp laceration repair algorithm:

1. Inspect the wound for foreign bodies and injury to the galea, and obtain as much hemostasis as possible by holding direct pressure over the wound (one or two fingers).
2. Apply topical lidocaine-epinephrine-tetracaine compound gel for anesthesia for wounds greater than 2 cm and for pediatric patients in significant distress, allowing 15–20 min for adequate depth of anesthesia. For wounds less than 2 cm you can proceed to Step 3. I have found that placement of less than two staples causes minimal distress even to very young patients. Topically applied LET gel results in adequate anesthesia of the epidermis prior to closure with stainless steel staples. Application of topical anesthesia will not result in additional trauma to and hemorrhage from the wound.
3. Cleanse the wound with three iodine/iodine swabs moving in a circle from wound edge to about 1–2 cm outward.

4. Using sterile pickups with teeth, evert and align the wound edges. Place surgical stapler flush with the skin so staples insert at a 90° angle and then deploy staples. Place one staple per centimeter of wound.
5. Finally apply a small amount of bacitracin to the wound. Patients can be allowed to wash their hair with mild shampoo and gently towel dry 1–2 days after wound closure. Patients can even be allowed to swim with this type of closure.
6. Remove the staples after 7–10 days.

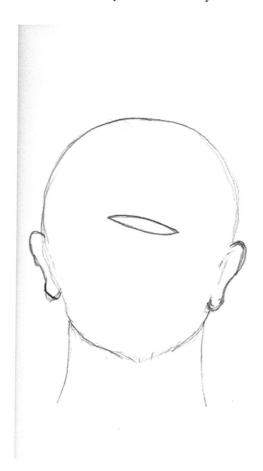

Scalp laceration

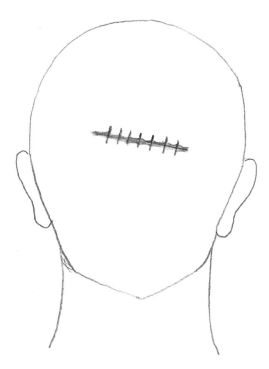

Scalp laceration repaired with staples

## 7.2 Face

Proper repair of facial lacerations can be difficult, especially in young children or
others in significant distress. If you feel at all uncomfortable, then refer the patient
to a local Emergency Department with an ENT or plastic surgery team on call or at
least with the ability to perform pediatric sedation.

As in the scalp, there are multiple tissue layers in the face to be aware of when
repairing a laceration to this anatomic area. The superficial muscular aponeurotic
system (SMAS) is an extension of the platysma muscle of the neck that connects
with the galea over the frontalis muscle. Similar to scalp lacerations, injuries to the
SMAS, which lies just below the epidermis, should be repaired to prevent spreading
of the wound and weakness of the muscles of facial expression.

Prior to suturing a facial laceration, topical anesthetic compound cream or gel
should be applied (LET, LAT, or EMLA). This has been found to improve patient satisfaction and decrease patient discomfort [33]. If the patient is more comfortable, it is
also easier for the provider to provide optimal care and closure of the wound.

For improved cosmesis and decreased inflammatory response, all facial lacerations should be closed with a 6-0 or 7-0 suture. For children it is preferable to use a
6-0 fast-absorbing chromic gut so that you do not have to remove the sutures later.
This results in improved patient emotional and physical comfort with the procedure

[34]. As discussed previously, Vicryl suture should not be utilized in epidermal closure as it causes increased inflammation, which can lead to localized granuloma formation and scarring. Monocryl buried suture would also be a poorer choice in a contaminated wound as this can increase the chance of infection.

Lacerations involving a mucosal surface can be approximated using 5-0 chromic gut, which will dissolve in about 7–10 days. If this suture is not available, Vicryl can be used inside of the mouth, although it will take significantly longer to dissolve than chromic gut (14–20 days).

Tissue adhesive (butylcyanoacrylate or octylcyanoacrylate) may be utilized in closure of acute facial lacerations. Advantages of tissue adhesive include ease of application, minimal patient discomfort, and cosmetic outcome equal to sutured repair in randomized controlled trials [35]. To optimize outcomes in the use of tissue adhesives, wounds should be acute (<12 h old), linear, under no tension, and hemostatic. Wounds under tension will spread resulting in poor cosmesis and wide scar formation. There are also no currently published studies evaluating the safety and efficacy of using tissue adhesives on the lip or mucosal surfaces. Disadvantages may include children biting, licking, or sucking on the glue leading to dehiscence, potential toxicity, and inadequate cosmesis of the vermillion border [36].

Finally, when repairing a facial laceration, use as many sutures as is necessary to get a tight closure of the wound, especially at the corners. Any gapping or spreading of the wound will result in a widening of the scar. The wound should be approximated with very small (1–2 mm) bites to prevent inversion of the skin edges.

The following sections contain references for repairing lacerations of specific regions of the face using sutures.

### 7.2.1 Eyebrow

When addressing a laceration that occurs vertically through the brow, it is important to line up the superior and inferior hairlines before infiltrating with anesthetic (which will distort the brow architecture). Failure to do so will result in a very visible deformity of the brow.

1. Find the superior medial and superior lateral edge of the hairline and mark with a sterile marking pen. Then do the same on the inferior medial and inferior lateral edges.
2. Cleanse with three iodine swipes. Do not use chlorhexidine near the eye region as it can get in the eyes and cause injury.
3. Infiltrate with an adequate amount of lidocaine with epinephrine (usually 1–2 cm$^3$).
4. Start re-approximating the superior and then inferior brow edges and then bisecting the remaining incision until you have full approximation, taking care near the corners to prevent gapping.
5. Apply bacitracin and a sterile dressing that can be removed in 2 days.
6. Sutures should be removed in 5 days to prevent excessive scarring.

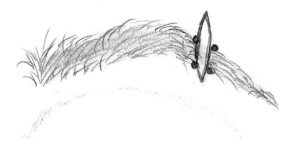

Eyebrow laceration

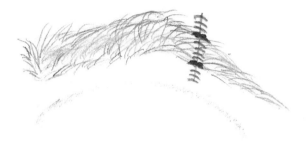

Eyebrow laceration repaired with green simple interrupted suture

## 7.2.2  Ear

The ear is composed of a cartilaginous skeleton with tightly adherent skin. Lacerations can be simple, involving skin only, or complex, involving skin and cartilage.

1. Cleanse the skin around the wound with chlorhexidine prior to infiltrating with anesthetic.
2. Infiltrate the wound with adequate lidocaine to anesthetize the wound. *Do not use Epinephrine on the ear.* This can result in necrosis of the skin and poorly vascularized cartilage.
3. Inspect the wound for damage to the cartilage or perichondral hematoma. Any ragged edges of cartilage should be carefully debrided (no more than 5 mm). If there is a perichondral hematoma, incision should be made within the curve of the helix or antihelix to hide scarring, and the hematoma should be carefully evacuated from the perichondral space to prevent damage to the cartilage.

4. Close the skin over the cartilage by taking small bites and moving around the outside of the helix to the posterior skin or closing in two layers (anterior and posterior) for through and through lacerations. Do not attempt to repair tears in the cartilage as it is weak, poorly vascularized, and does not hold suture well.
5. Following repair of an ear laceration, it is important to place an adequate compression dressing over the ear to prevent a hematoma from forming. Failure to drain or prevent perichondral hematoma can result in necrosis and scar tissue known as "cauliflower ear." A compression dressing is made by first placing a small amount of petrolatum gauze (Xeroform) within the canal and over the wound. Then take a large amount of sterile gauze and place it behind and in front of the auricle. Finally wrap the head and ear tightly with gauze or Coban. This dressing can be removed in 48 h.
6. Sutures can be removed in 5–7 days.

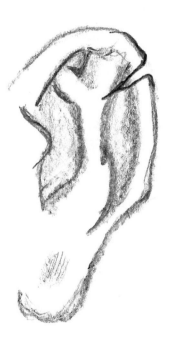
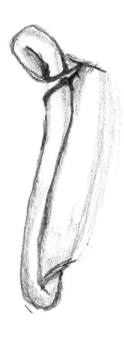

Ear laceration (through and through)

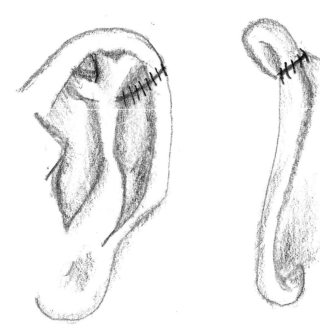

Ear laceration repaired with simple interrupted sutures

### 7.2.3 Nose

Injuries to the nose are similar to injuries to the ear, but unlike the ear, through and through injuries should not be addressed in the urgent care and should be sent to an Emergency Department with an ENT or plastic surgery specialist on call.

1. Cleanse the skin around the wound with iodine or chlorhexidine after evaluating for any injuries to the cartilage that should be treated by a specialist. Also if any force was encountered during the trauma, inspect the septum for a septal hematoma. Like a preauricular hematoma, this must be drained to prevent pressure necrosis of the cartilage and mucosa of the septum.
2. Infiltrate the wound with an adequate amount of lidocaine. (Do not use epinephrine as it can result in necrosis of the poorly vascularized skin and cartilage.)
3. Repair the epidermal lacerations only.
4. Apply bacitracin and a sterile dressing that can be removed in 5 days.
5. Remove the sutures in 5 days.

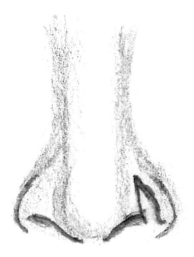

Nose laceration

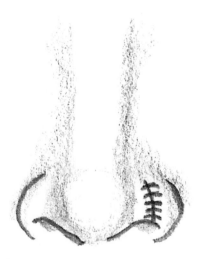

Nose laceration repaired with simple interrupted sutures

## 7.2.4   Lip

There are several unique aspects of the anatomy of the lip that will need to be evaluated prior to repair. One is proper re-approximation of the vermillion border, another is through and through injury, and the final is repair of the mucosa.

1. Inspect the wound carefully. If there is injury through the muscle of the orbicularis oris, do not attempt to repair this wound and send the patient to an Emergency Department with a facial specialist. Improper closure of this muscle can result in difficult speaking, chewing, and making facial expressions.

2. If there is injury through the vermillion border of the lip, this should be addressed in the same fashion as a vertical eyebrow laceration. Prior to infiltration with anesthetic, mark the medial and lateral edge of the vermillion very precisely with a sterile marking pen. Even a millimeter of error will be very visible to the patient in this delicate region.

3. Cleanse the skin around the wound with three iodine swabs as chlorhexidine in the concentrated form is toxic and should never be used to cleanse around or in the mouth.

4. Infiltrate the wound with an adequate amount of lidocaine with or without epinephrine.

5. Approximate the vermilion border first and then bisect the remainder of the wound using small bites and closely spaced sutures. For the epithelial surfaces, 6-0 nylon or prolene is adequate. For any mucosal surfaces, use 5-0 or 6-0 chromic gut.

6. Do not apply any antibiotic ointment, as bacitracin is harmful if swallowed. You can offer the patient a non-antibiotic ointment like Aquaphor, if available.

7. Remove sutures in 5 days, except for mucosal sutures, which will dissolve in 7–10 days.

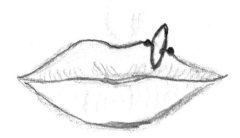

Lip laceration (through vermillion border)

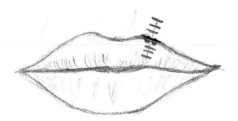

Lip laceration repaired with simple interrupted sutures

### 7.2.5  Other Facial Regions

1. Cleanse the region with iodine or chlorhexidine depending on proximity to the eye or mouth.
2. Infiltrate with an adequate amount of lidocaine with or without epinephrine.
3. Identify and repair any injuries to the SMAS with 5-0 Vicryl sutures. One indicator of injury to the SMAS would be a wound that is widened and difficult to approximate or that the wound appears to be under tension. Grasping just below the dermis, you should encounter a sturdy facial layer, which is the SMAS. Lacerations of the chin and forehead are regions where this is most commonly encountered.
4. Re-approximate the skin by bisecting the wound, making sure to use closely spaced 6-0 nylon or prolene simple interrupted sutures and taking small bites (1–2 mm from the skin edge).
5. Apply bacitracin and a sterile dressing that can be removed in 2 days.
6. Remove sutures in 5 days.

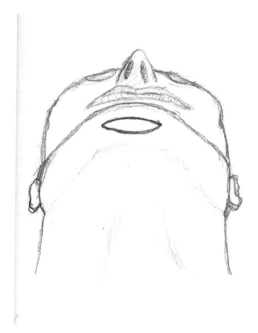

Chin laceration

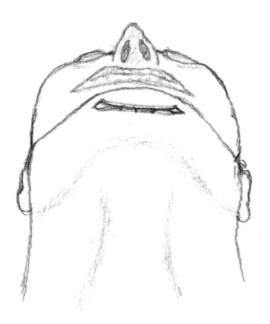

Chin laceration with SMAS repaired with interrupted buried dissolvable sutures

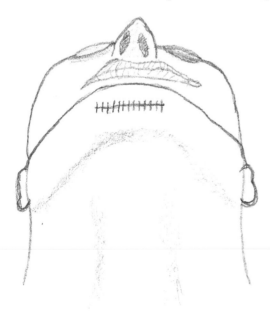

Chin laceration repaired with simple interrupted sutures

## 7.3  Neck and Trunk

It should be relatively rare that you encounter injuries to the neck and trunk in the urgent care setting. Be sure to thoroughly examine any wounds in these regions for muscle violation. If a wound passes through muscle, there is a much higher chance of concurrent devastating injury. If you encounter a wound like this in the urgent care setting, immediately transport the patient to the nearest Emergency Department via ambulance. Prior to transport, these wounds can be irrigated and packed with moist sterile gauze to prevent wound desiccation; however, this should not hinder expeditious transport to a higher level of care.

For superficial wounds of the neck and trunk, a method similar to facial wound re-approximation will be employed. A subcutaneous fascia lies between the skin and the fascial muscle layer on most parts of the body (neck, trunk, arms and legs). This subcutaneous fascia is composed of two layers, the fatty layer and the elastic layer. When preparing to repair wounds of the neck, trunk, and extremities, this layer should be identified. Use caution – be sure that you can grasp the elastic layer with the forceps before placing any dissolvable sutures in this layer. If you place sutures into the fatty tissue, they will cause damage and necrosis, which can increase the likelihood of deep space infections.

### 7.3.1  Repairing Superficial Neck and Trunk Lacerations

1. Cleanse the skin around the wound with iodine or chlorhexidine.
2. Infiltrate with an adequate amount of lidocaine with or without epinephrine.
3. Identify and repair any injuries to the subcutaneous fascia with 4-0 Vicryl sutures. One indicator of injury to the subcutaneous fascia would be a wound that is widened and difficult to approximate or a wound under tension. Grasping just below the dermis, you should encounter a sturdy facial layer, which is the elastic layer of the subcutaneous fascia.
4. Re-approximate the skin by bisecting the wound, making sure to use closely spaced 5-0 nylon or prolene simple interrupted sutures and taking small bites (1–2 mm from the skin edge).

   I recommend 4-0 nylon or prolene for the thickened posterior dermis. In addition, for wounds on the posterior neck and back, I would recommend a vertical or horizontal mattress suture technique over a simple interrupted suture technique. This is because the skin in this region tends to be under greater tension, especially on concave surfaces. The horizontal mattress suture technique releases some of the pressure from the wound edges and also everts the epidermal edges to allow better approximation. Eversion can be obtained with simple interrupted suturing alone and tends to be operator dependent.

5. Apply bacitracin and a sterile dressing that can be removed in 2 days.
6. Remove sutures in 7–10 days.

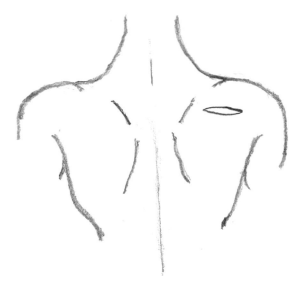

Shoulder laceration

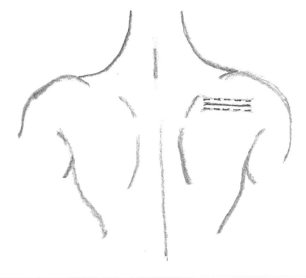

Shoulder laceration repaired with horizontal mattress sutures

## 7.4   Upper Extremity

Wounds of the upper extremity (arms, hands, fingers) are by far the most common wounds that you will evaluate in the urgent care. Overall these wounds are simple to approximate, but several situations require special attention including wounds over a joint, open fractures, and wounds under tension.

### *7.4.1   Repair of Lacerations to the Arm*

Wounds of the arm will likely include wounds to the subcutaneous fascia and should be treated in a similar fashion to wounds of the neck and trunk. Wounds over the elbow should be thoroughly evaluated for violation of the joint or bursa. If you do not have the ability to perform saline arthrogram (this technique will not be explained in this text as I don't believe it should be performed by someone without proper training), then you should triage these patients to the ED for orthopedic evaluation.

1. Cleanse the skin around the wound with iodine or chlorhexidine.
2. Infiltrate the skin and deeper tissues with an adequate amount of lidocaine with or without epinephrine.
3. Identify and repair any injuries to the subcutaneous fascia with 4-0 or 5-0 Vicryl sutures. Grasping just below the dermis, you should encounter a sturdy facial layer, which is the elastic layer of the subcutaneous fascia.
4. Re-approximate the skin by bisecting the wound, making sure to use closely spaced 5-0 nylon or prolene simple interrupted sutures and taking small bites (1–2 mm from the skin edge).

    (a) Wounds to the elbow that do not involve the joint can be approximated using the vertical mattress technique to provide additional reinforcement against tension created when flexing at the elbow. If you have difficulty approximating a wound of the elbow without tension using the vertical mattress suturing technique, I would recommend a stapled closure. This is very durable at this location and does not result in an increased likelihood of unsightly scarring.

    (b) Wounds of the volar forearm should be closed using the horizontal mattress suture technique. This lessens the tension over the surface of a wound on a convex or flexion surface, including the wrist.

    (c) Skin tears on the elderly that can be easily approximated without tension should be treated with tissue glue to prevent undue tension on fragile skin. Do not attempt to approximate a skin tear that is already adherent or under tension. Best practice and clinical evidence in the treatment of skin tears can be found in the chapter dedicated to these specialized wounds.

5. Apply bacitracin and a sterile dressing that can be removed in 2 days.
6. Remove sutures in 7 days.

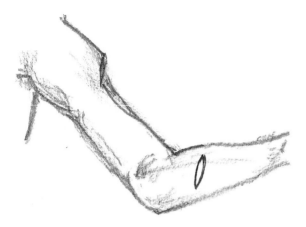

Forearm laceration

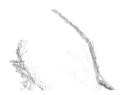

Forearm laceration repaired with horizontal mattress sutures

### 7.4.2  Hands and Fingers

Wounds of the hands and fingers are very similar to those of the arm with one key difference; there is no subcutaneous fascia in this location. For this reason, never attempt to place deep sutures into the hand or fingers. Bleeding should be controlled with a temporary tourniquet, followed by a closure and a pressure dressing. Do not attempt to place a suture ligature around bleeding vessels. This can lead to distal necrosis and increased likelihood of infection.

1. Cleanse the entire digit with iodine or chlorhexidine.
2. In the hand local anesthetic can be directly infiltrated around the wound as in other locations using lidocaine either with or without epinephrine. For digital anesthesia, it is preferable to perform a ring block for anesthesia using 2 % lidocaine without epinephrine.

   A ring block is obtained by inserting the needle through the skin proximal to the injury, on the lateral aspect of the finger, perpendicular to the bone. When the bone is encountered, retract the needle slightly, and infiltrate anesthetic in three directions: along the nerve, dorsal to the bone, and palmar to the bone. This technique is then repeated on the medial side of the finger to anesthetize both digital nerves.

3. Re-approximate the skin by bisecting the wound, making sure to use closely spaced 5-0 nylon or prolene simple interrupted sutures and taking small bites (1–2 mm from the skin edge).

   (a) For the palm of the hand, I recommend using the horizontal mattress suturing technique to lessen tension on wound edges when flexing and extending the fingers.
   (b) Webspaces should also be approximated using the horizontal mattress suturing technique for the same reasons.

4. Apply bacitracin and a sterile dressing that can be removed in 2 days. Wounds to the fingers that directly involve a joint can be splinted for the first 2 days to facilitate the initial epidermal closure. Avoid prolonged splinting, however, which can lead to joint stiffness and immobility after a period of only 3–5 days.
5. Remove sutures in 10 days.

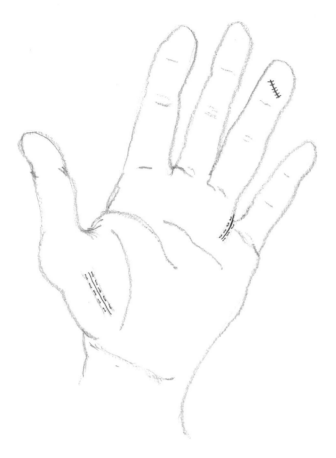

Three repairs of hand lacerations: distal fingertip repaired with simple interrupted sutures, webspace repaired with horizontal mattress sutures, and palm repaired with horizontal mattress sutures

## 7.5   Lower Extremity

Treatment of wounds of the upper extremity and lower extremity are for the most part similar. Like the elbow injuries to the knee should be evaluated for violation of the joint and bursa. If you are not capable of performing a saline arthrogram, then these wounds should be triaged to an ED with orthopedic capabilities.

### 7.5.1   *Upper Leg*

These wounds are very similar to those found on the upper extremities and trunk and can be treated in a similar fashion.

1. Cleanse the skin around the wound with iodine or chlorhexidine.
2. Infiltrate with an adequate amount of lidocaine with or without epinephrine.
3. Identify and repair any injuries to the subcutaneous fascia with 4-0 Vicryl sutures. Grasping just below the dermis, you should encounter a sturdy facial layer, which is the elastic layer of the subcutaneous fascia.
4. Re-approximate the skin by bisecting the wound, making sure to use closely spaced 5-0 nylon or prolene horizontal mattress sutures and taking small bites (1–2 mm from the skin edge). On the upper thigh, most regions will be convex in nature, and a horizontal mattress suture can provide additional buttressing of these wounds to prevent widening under tension.
5. Apply bacitracin and a sterile dressing that can be removed in 2 days.
6. Remove sutures in 7–10 days.

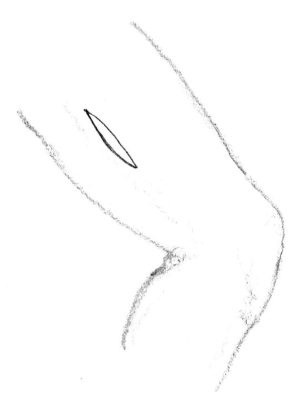

Upper leg laceration

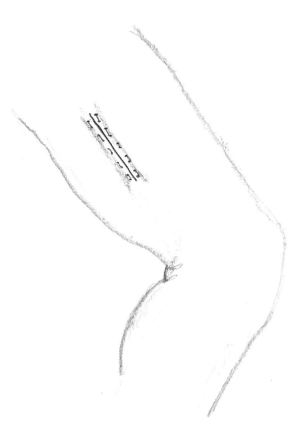

Upper leg laceration repaired with horizontal mattress sutures

## 7.5.2   Lower Leg (From the Knee Down)

The skin and subcutaneous fascia of the lower leg is densely adherent to the under-lying muscle fascia and can be very difficult to approximate without undue tension. If not treated properly, these wounds can dehisce, necessitating long-term wound treatment and closure by secondary intention. This is also true for wounds overlying the knee, which are subject to significant stress during ambulation and other daily activities. For this reason, I recommend closing all wounds from the knee to the ankle with stainless steel staples. There has been some hesitancy to utilize staples in orthopedic surgery, as there was a concern for increase in wound infection. This was found to be true only for hip arthroplasty and the difference was minimal. Overall there was no significant difference in dehiscence, discharge, skin necrosis, scarring, or inflammation between the stapling and suturing in orthopedic surgery [37].

1. Cleanse the skin around the wound with iodine or chlorhexidine.
2. Infiltrate with an adequate amount of lidocaine with or without epinephrine.
3. Identify any adhesions to the muscle fascia that may need to be dissected in order to bring the epidermal edges into approximation. This can be done by gently snipping below the surface of the dermis with a sharp tissue scissors.
4. Once the epidermal edges can be approximated without tension, close the skin by bisecting the wound, using stainless steel staples. This may require assistance from a medical assistant, nurse, or other medical professionals to evert the edges with forceps while you place the staples.
5. Apply bacitracin and a sterile dressing that can be removed in 2 days. Do not splint the knee joint. This will lead to undue stiffness of the joint, possibly necessitating physical therapy intervention following wound healing.
6. Remove staples in 10 days.

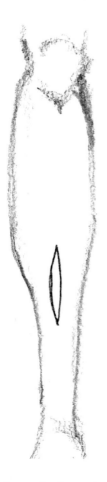

Lower leg laceration

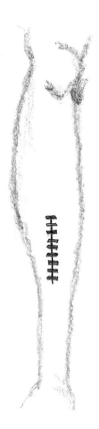

Lower leg laceration repaired with staples

## 7.5.3  *Feet and Toes*

Wounds of the feet and toes are very similar to those of the hand and fingers. Never attempt to place deep sutures into the foot or toes. Bleeding should be controlled with a temporary tourniquet, followed by a closure and a pressure dressing. No not attempt to place a suture ligature around bleeding vessels. This can lead to distal necrosis and increased likelihood of infection.

1. Cleanse the entire digit with iodine or chlorhexidine.
2. In the hand local anesthetic can be directly infiltrated around the wound as in other locations using lidocaine either with or without epinephrine. For digital

anesthesia, it is preferable to perform a ring block for anesthesia using 2 % lido-caine without epinephrine.

A ring block is obtained by inserting the needle through the skin proximal to the injury, on the lateral aspect of the toe perpendicular to the bone. When the bone is encountered, retract the needle slightly, and infiltrate anesthetic in three directions: along the nerve, dorsal to the bone, and palmar to the bone. This technique is then repeated on the medial side of the toe to anesthetize both digital nerves.

3. Re-approximate the skin by bisecting the wound, making sure to use closely spaced 5-0 nylon or prolene simple interrupted sutures and taking small bites (1–2 mm from the skin edge).

   (a) For the plantar surface of the foot, I recommend using the horizontal mat-tress suturing technique to lessen tension on wound edges when ambulating.
   (b) Webspaces should also be approximated using the horizontal mattress sutur-ing technique for the same reasons.

4. Apply bacitracin and a sterile dressing that can be removed in 2 days. Wounds to the fingers that directly involve a joint can be splinted for the first 2 days to facili-tate the initial epidermal closure. Avoid prolonged splinting, however, which can lead to joint stiffness and immobility after a period of only 3–5 days.
5. Remove sutures in 10 days.

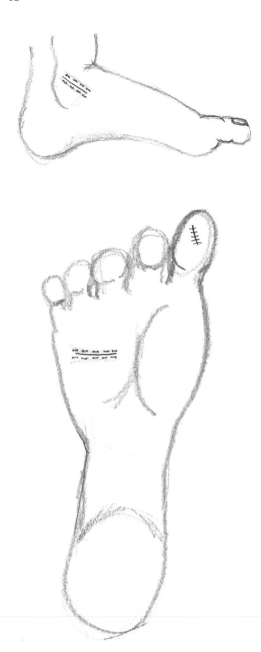

Three repairs of foot lacerations: lateral ankle repaired with horizontal mattress sutures, distal toe repaired with simple interrupted sutures, and plantar surface repaired with horizontal mattress sutures

# Chapter 8
# Special Circumstances in Wounds

There are types of wounds in which closure with primary intention is not possible or the best option. When confronted with these types of wounds in the urgent care, a provider should have a basic knowledge of how to provide immediate treatment of the wound so that the patient can be referred back to their primary care physician or a referral can be made to the appropriate wound care specialist. These wounds include skin avulsion of the elderly (skin tears), wounds in edematous patients, vascular and/or diabetic ulcers, and burns.

## 8.1 Skin Tears in the Elderly

Skin avulsions or skin tears are very common in an aging population. Yearly estimate of skin tear prevalence in an institutionalized population is about 1.5 million skin tears per year, with even more in the ambulatory population unaccounted for. The 1993 study by Payne and Martin defined a skin tear as "a traumatic wound occurring principally on the extremities of older adults, as a result of shearing or friction forces which separate the epidermis from the dermis (partial thickness wound) or which separate the epidermis and the dermis from underlying structures (full thickness wound) [38]." Often minor trauma, such as hitting a leg or arm on a wall, door, or car door, or even the act of being assisted by a caretaker, results in significant separation of the epidermis and dermis from the underlying tissue. Skin tears cause a significant amount of morbidity in an elderly population, and for a long time, there was a lack of evidence-based care algorithms. Because of this an international advisory council on skin tears was established to provide prevention and treatment guidelines for the management of skin tears and facilitate a best practice management system. For this reason the STAR classification was developed and validated in 2006, but it wasn't until 2011 that a universal definition and global comprehensive strategy was established [39].

© Springer International Publishing Switzerland 2016
B. Busse, *Wound Management in Urgent Care*,
DOI 10.1007/978-3-319-27428-7_8

## 8.1.1  Risk Factors Associated with Skin Tears

There are several modifiable and non-modifiable risk factors related to aging that result in increased fragility of the skin. It is important to recognize these risk factors among an aging patient population in your assessment. When it comes to skin tears, prevention is tantamount to treatment.

Comorbid disease, poor vascularity, and inadequate collagen repair and replacement can lead to thinning and weakening of the skin as we age.

There is loss of dermal and subcutaneous tissue due to decreased production of collagen, as well as epidermal thinning, and flattening of the dermal/epidermal junction [40, 41]. A combination of these and other factors leads to a loss of elasticity as well as tensile strength leading to intrinsic weakening of the epidermal and dermal attachments. Because of this, the epidermis can be more easily separated from the underlying dermis or hypodermis.

A second risk factor to loss of epidermal integrity is drying of the skin. Elderly persons have a reduced amount of sebum production due to decreases in the number and activity of sebaceous glands [41, 42]. Drying of the skin is further exacerbated by the need for frequent washing, alkaline soaps, and, in the colder months of the year, evaporation when homes are heated with dry heat. It is important to educate patients on the importance of daily use of moisturizers, especially those that do not contain alcohol, which can actually lead to additional dryness over time.

Another known risk factor for developing skin tears is ecchymosis and/or hematoma of the skin. Frequently, medications taken for anticoagulation to prevent strokes and myocardial infarctions lead to the development of multiple ecchymosis. These areas are at increased risk for tearing when subjected to friction. As an urgent care provider, you may recommend older patients that you evaluate with multiple ecchymosis to request a referral for a home safety evaluation from their primary care provider, or you may be able to send out the referral yourself.

In addition many intrinsic factors of an elderly population increase their propensity for developing skin tears including: impaired balance and mobility, impaired vision, dehydration, poor nutrition, and decreased sensation. Because of the need for increased assistance, persons with impairment have a greater risk for shear, friction, and blunt force injuries compared to those without impairments. Oftentimes, those requiring the most care are those most at risk for accidental trauma resulting in skin tears [43].

As a physician, it is important that your interactions with elderly patients improve their quality of life, and a few simple interventions can reduce patient risk of skin tears. Counseling patients on smoking cessation to improve blood flow and circulation is an important piece of caring for the elderly. In addition, nutrition and hydration counseling should be undertaken at every visit. Home safety evaluations can be a critical part of risk detection and reduction as mentioned above. In addition, as a care provider, you should reevaluate prescribing medications to elderly patients that could further impair their balance and coordination leading to injury.

## 8.2   Evidence-Based Approach to Caring for Skin Tears

The following will guide you through the assessment and management of skin tears using an evidence-based approach; however, each person's case can be addressed individually to provide optimal healing and management based on their unique physiology and comorbid diseases.

### 8.2.1   Wound Assessment

Before beginning you should attempt to get adequate control of any bleeding occurring at the wound site. Next, an attempt should be made to realign the flap with the wound bed. Wound assessment of skin tears can then be undertaken using the STAR (Skin Tear Audit Research) tools [44].

- *Category 1a*: A skin tear where the edges can be realigned in the normal anatomical position (without undue tension) and the flap color is not pale, dusky, or darkened
- *Category 1b*: A skin tear where the edges can be realigned in the normal anatomical position (without undue tension) and the flap is pale, dusky, or darkened
- *Category 2a*: A skin flap where the edges cannot be realigned in the normal anatomical position and the flap is not pale, dusky, or darkened
- *Category 2b*: A skin flap where the edges cannot be realigned in the normal anatomical position and the flap is pale, dusky, or darkened
- *Category 3*: A skin tear where the flap is completely absent

### 8.2.2   Skin Cleansing and Wound Preparation

As with other types of traumatic wounds, the wound bed needs to be cleansed of any dirt, debris, slough, or bacterial biofilms to optimize wound healing to prevent infections [45].

Wound cleansing should be done gently with normal saline (again avoiding the use of iodine or chlorhexidine on the wound surface which can be toxic to the granulation tissue and impair wound healing). For areas with large amounts of contamination and stuck-on debris, the wound can be cleansed using a piston syringe and either splatter shield or 19G angiocatheter to force the water out under pressure at about 8 psi.

Two contradictory actions must be taken at this point: preservation of as much of the skin flap as possible and removal of any nonviable skin which may impede wound healing. For this reason any frankly necrotic skin should be carefully trimmed. This can be a difficult assessment when it comes to skin tears, as many areas of the wound may appear dusky, darkened, or discolored. Torn, very thin, or rolled-up edges of epidermis should be carefully trimmed away on the skin flap pedicle to portions of healthy dermis with a bleeding edge. If the skin viability is questionable, it is better to leave it intact rather than to trim away too much skin.

## 8.2.3   Treatment

The consensus statements on skin tear management recommend moist wound healing in all cases of skin tear treatment [39].

Given the fragility of elderly skin as discussed above, closure with primary intention (sutures or staples) is not viable or recommended. The skin can further tear away from the sutures and may result in additional loss of tenuous skin. One study recommended the use of skin adhesive tapes over the use of sutures or staples. The validity of this research has since been disproven as skin adhesive tapes can result in epidermal shearing and injury especially if not properly removed [46].

The first principal of wound healing for skin tears is to create a moist environment. Epidermal cells and other cells necessary to restore skin integrity are best able to function in a moist environment.

The Registered Nurses Association of Ontario and Ovington and Pierce have outlined several key factors for the treatment of skin tears:

1. Maintain constant moisture
2. Suit the local wound environment
3. Protect the periwound skin
4. Control and manage exudates
5. Control and manage infection
6. Optimize caregiver time

### 8.2.3.1   Type 1 Wounds (Those with Adequate Approximation)

Type 1a/b wounds can be repaired using 2-octyl cyanoacrylate topical tissue adhesive. Recent literature supports this recommendation with complete closure seen in only one application of adhesive, with no reported wound infections [46, 47].

### 8.2.3.2   Type 2 and 3 Wounds (Those with >25 % Skin Loss)

The most common wound dressing that can be used in Category 2a/b wound will be an alginate or lipo-colloid mesh with successful healing described in 7–10 days in optimal conditions [48]. Segments of the dressing should be carefully trimmed and applied to the wound bed without overlapping the intact epidermis of the periwound area. This protects the periwound from maceration and injury.

After application of the moist dressing, the wound can be carefully wrapped with gauze or a gentle pressure dressing (ACE compression wrap or Coban). Be careful to avoid excessive pressure, which can impair blood flow to the healing tissues. Never place adhesive tapes or clear adhesive dressings onto the skin of elderly patients with skin tears. Like adhesive wound closure strips, improper removal of adhesive tapes and dressings can lead to additional epidermal stripping and skin injury.

## 8.3  Bite Wounds

Mammalian bite wounds are very common and account for nearly 2 % of all emergency room/urgent care visits. Bite wounds are a special type of wound that needs to be addressed differently than acute wounds from other cutting/piercing trauma. Due to the extent and type of bacterial contamination, these wounds are at a high risk for cellulitis and deep soft tissue infection.

Risk of infection can correlate with the species that inflicted the bite wound with cat bites resulting in the most infections, followed by human bites and then dog bites. Wound characteristics that predispose to infection include deep puncture wounds, wounds with a large amount of tissue destruction, wounds in areas of edema or hypoperfusion, wounds near a joint, or wounds of the hands, feet, face, or genitals. Because depth of wound is more important than wound severity, wounds that may appear innocuous may result in severe infection. This is especially true for cat bites, which involve small punctures with very deep penetration. Patients with impaired immunity either due to illness, extremes of age (<2 or >65), or immuno-suppressant medications are also at greater risk for infection.

### 8.3.1  Dog and Cat Bite Treatment

**Bite Wound Treatment**
- Anesthetize
- Explore
- Irrigate
- Debride
- Close

Most animal bites are inflicted by an animal who is familiar to the patient, either their own or belonging to someone close to them. Bites can be graded on a scale from 1 to 4 based on the depth of injury from superficial to deep muscle and/or nerve, blood vessels, or bone [49].

Patients with animal bites should be evaluated in a systematic manner similar to patients with other traumatic injury. Patients with concern for, or evidence of, joint, bone, tendon, or nerve/blood vessel damage should be triaged to the Emergency Department. Patients presenting with signs of uncontrolled hemorrhage or shock should be stabilized and transported via ambulance to an Emergency Department. Once patients are determined stable, then further treatment is initiated. First the injured area should be appropriately anesthetized with lidocaine with or without epinephrine. Once adequate anesthesia is administered, the wound should be explored to determine the depth and tissues affected. Following exploration, the wound should be copiously irrigated with 200–500 mL of normal saline using a syringe and 19 gauge angiocatheter. All devitalized, crushed, and/or necrotic tissue should be removed from the wound. Previous practice standards accepted that all facial wounds should be closed primarily [50] and limb wounds left to heal by secondary intention.

Current research shows, however, that limb wounds up to 12 h old that are repaired primarily do not have any greater risk of infection than those left to heal by secondary intention [51].

**Risk Factors for Infection of Animal Bites**
- Deep wounds of the hands, feet, joints, face, or genitals
- Wounds in patients with edema or impaired circulation
- Patients at risk for infection (elderly, infant, immunocompromised)
- Patients with implants

Prophylaxis against infection is not universally recommended based on the evidence, except in high-risk cases [52]. Antibiotics are not recommended for wounds greater than 24 h old, not presenting with signs of infection [53]. Animal bites are typically mixed aerobic and anaerobic type infections [54]. For dog and cat bites, the most commonly cultured organisms are *Pasteurella multocida*, *Staphylococcus* sp. (including MRSA), alpha-hemolytic *Streptococcus*, *Actinomyces*, and *Fusobacterium* [55]. A broad-spectrum antibiotic like amoxicillin-clavulanate 875/125 mg PO every 12 h or clindamycin 300 mg PO every 8 h plus a fluoroquinolone (ciprofloxacin 500 mg PO every 12 h or levofloxacin 750 mg PO every day or moxifloxacin 400 mg PO every day) [56] is adequate for prophylaxis for most dog bite injuries. *Pasteurella multocida* has been shown to be resistant to clindamycin monotherapy, as well as macrolides, aminoglycosides, and group 1 cephalosporins. This therapy can be discontinued after 3–5 days provided there are not ongoing signs of cellulitis or deep tissue infection. Signs of cellulitis and/or soft tissue infection can include redness, swelling, purulence, pain of the tissues surrounding the bite, fevers, and/or malaise. For patients presenting with cellulitis, antibiotics should be continued for 7–14 days, 2–3 weeks for tenosynovitis, and 3–4 weeks for osteomyelitis [55]. Patients presenting with systemic signs of infection (fever, malaise, tachycardia, hypotension) should be triaged to the Emergency Department. All bites should receive tetanus prophylaxis.

### 8.3.2  Human Bite Treatment

Human bites are usually found in an oval configuration for intentional bites or can be indirect from contact of the fist to the mouth during an altercation [57]. They are usually intentional and may signify child or domestic partner abuse. Although they may look innocuous on the surface, deep tissue injury and crush injury can occur with significant soft tissue damage and necrosis leading to infections.

Initial evaluation and treatment should proceed as with other mammalian bites. Once patients are determined stable, then further treatment is initiated. First the injured area should be appropriately anesthetized with lidocaine with or without epinephrine. Once adequate anesthesia is administered, the wound should be explored to determine the depth and tissues affected. Following exploration the wound should be copiously irrigated with 200–500 mL of normal saline using a syringe and 19G angiocatheter. All devitalized, crushed, and/or necrotic tissue should be removed from the wound. Primary closure of human bite wounds is only recommended in the treatment of cosmetically important facial wounds <24 h [58]. Non-facial human bite wounds, bites to the hand, and infected wounds should not be closed primarily [59].

Human bites contain very high densities of virulent and antibiotic-resistant bacteria including *Viridians streptococci*, *Staphylococcus aureus*, *Haemophilus influenzae*, and most importantly *Eikenella corrodens*. *Eikenella* is the pathogen most likely leading to infection of human bite wounds and is resistant to multiple antibiotics including clindamycin, erythromycin, anti-staphylococcal penicillins, aminoglycosides, and first-generation cephalosporins and should be treated with one dose parenteral cephalosporin if available and followed by amoxicillin-clavulanate 875/125 mg PO every 12 h for 3–5 days or clindamycin 300 mg PO every 8 h plus a fluoroquinolone (ciprofloxacin 500 mg PO every 12 h or levofloxacin 750 mg PO every day or moxifloxacin 400 mg PO every day) for 3–5 days for penicillin-allergic patients. If the patient presents with an already infected bite that is greater than 24 h old, they should be referred to the emergency room for appropriate therapy with parenteral antibiotics.

Human bites can also transfer pathologic viruses such as hepatitis B, hepatitis C, and HIV. It is currently recommended that patients with human bite wounds consider postexposure prophylaxis against HIV in high-risk cases or postexposure and 6-month follow-up testing [60]. All bites should receive tetanus prophylaxis.

## 8.4 Caring for Acute Wounds in Patients with Peripheral Edema

Patients may suffer from chronic limb edema due to a variety of conditions including congestive heart failure, congenital lymphedema, acquired lymph edema, or loss of lymphatic drainage secondary to oncologic procedures. Edema can also result naturally from acute severe wounding due to the processes of inflammation discussed earlier. In most cases that will be evaluated in the urgent care setting, this kind of edema should not play much of a role in wound healing, aside from the initial 2–3 days after wounding.

Patients with chronic edema may present to the urgent care with acute wounds from trauma, or they may present with chronic tissue breakdown. Chronic wounds and pressure wounds will be addressed in another chapter.

Chronic tissue edema has been shown to impair wound healing. In patients with normal flow of lymphatic fluid, the inflammatory fluid, protein, and cells that are released into the wound site at the time of injury are reabsorbed by the lymphatic channels, broken down, and recirculated into the bloodstream. The small valveless channels of the lymphatic system are present in the dermis and then join with larger vessels in the subdermal tissues. From here the larger, valved, lymphatic channels continue to bring the fluid centrally toward the lymph nodes and from there to the larger channels within the body, ending finally in the venous system. Chronic congestion of this system leads to impairment of drainage of lymphatic fluid and swelling of the peripheral tissues. The pressure of the edematous tissue impairs the ability of the body to initiate the wound healing cascade due to impaired capillary filling [61]. In addition plasma and other interstitial fluids will begin to leak through the disrupted epithelial and dermal layers leading to loss of epithelial integrity and delayed and/or incomplete wound healing. In most cases, management of injuries in patients with lymphedema will require prolonged and specialized treatment referred to as complex decompressive physiotherapy. This treatment involves long-term decompressive therapies as well as physical therapy to optimize lymphatic drainage and tissue healing at the site of injury.

In the urgent care setting, however, taking initial steps to provide optimal wound healing conditions and referring patients either directly to wound specialists or to their primary care physicians will optimize their wound healing outcomes.

1. Acute wounds in patients with lymphedema will likely not heal if approximated with suture, staples, glue, or adhesive strips, and the process of performing a primary closure can result in additional wounds and tissue trauma. When loss of epithelial integrity occurs in patients with chronic edema, it is difficult to reestablish, even under the best conditions, so when possible avoiding additional trauma in the effort to create a "closed" wound. If, however, wound re-approximation is necessary for wound hemostasis, it can be accomplished using few, widely spaced, simple interrupted sutures without undue tension. Edematous tissues typically have a loss of elasticity, and it is very important not to put tension on the wound, which may lead to necrosis and further tissue loss. Under most circumstances, avoid trying to close the wound with primary intention.

2. After cleansing is completed and you have adequate hemostasis, the skin can be gently approximated, and a moist dressing can be applied such as a lipo-alginate dressing. Avoid contact of the moist barrier dressing with intact epithelium, which can lead to maceration and tissue loss.

3. The most important aspect of wound care for a patient with lymph edema is compression. Apply large amounts of dry gauze to the wound to soak up excess fluid and then apply firm compression using either Coban dressing or an elastic bandage. Avoid applying so much pressure that you cause venous congestion distal to the wound (a reddish/purple hue distally).

4. The next key element of wound healing is keeping the wound as dry as possible. This will require frequent dressing changes in the initial period after wounding. If the patient cannot see their primary care doctor or wound specialist within 24 h, advise them to return daily for dressing changes until continuity of care can be established with a wound specialist.

Patients with chronic tissue edema can pose a challenge to all wound care specialist. Your goal in the urgent care setting is to help provide them with adequate wound dressing, compression, and expedient transfer of care to a wound specialist. Be sure the patient is aware of the increased need to keep the injured limb elevated as much as possible to keep the amount of drainage to a minimum. This is will help to improve the long-term outcomes of wound healing.

# Chapter 9
# Abscess Drainage

While abscess drainage may be thought of a fairly straightforward procedure, there are many nuances that should be addressed in the assessment and aftercare of patients with abscess.

When assessing a potential abscess for drainage, one should consider the size and location of the abscess as well as the potential for chronic disease at that location. The patient should be questioned as to prior history of abscess at the same location or other locations, history of MRSA (methicillin-resistant *Staphylococcus aureus*), hospitalizations (increasing the risk for potential MRSA infection), history of drug abuse, and past medical history (especially concerning immune impairment, presence of diabetes, or immunosuppressive drug therapy). This information can help you to determine the best course of action concerning whether or not to prescribe post-procedure antibiotic therapy, which is typically unnecessary in young healthy patients with limited prior history [62]. Antibiotics may be prescribed in those with impaired immunity, the elderly, and patients with history of MRSA.

An abscess will typically present as a fluctuant, painful nodule with surrounding induration and erythema representing inflammation and cellulitis. There may or may not be visible purulence beneath the surface of the skin or a draining punctum. If the patient presents with a potential abscess that is already draining or with a purulent punctum, then formal incision and drainage can typically be deferred for a period of 2–5 days, depending on the severity of surrounding inflammation and patient tolerance of the pain caused by the lesion. Soaking in warm water with Epsom salt or dilute hydrogen peroxide is typically recommended for 15 min every 2–12 h (depending on the location and the patient's ability to comply with the time period prescribed—for instance, a paronychia may be soaked more frequently than an abscess of the upper thigh). The extent of inflammation (erythema) should be marked on the patient's skin, and the patient should be instructed to return if the erythema extended more than 2 cm outside of the marked border.

© Springer International Publishing Switzerland 2016
B. Busse, *Wound Management in Urgent Care*,
DOI 10.1007/978-3-319-27428-7_9

If a patient presents with systemic signs of infection (fevers, tachycardia, hypotension), a referral to the Emergency Department is warranted as localized infection, like abscesses, typically does not cause systemic symptoms and these symptoms may represent progression to bacteremia or a necrotizing infection.

Another physical exam finding that would necessitate referral to the emergency room would be the presence of a pulsation at or near the site of abscess. Any pulsatile masses or abscess of the neck should not be incised in the clinic and should be referred to the nearest Emergency Department for further assessment.

Finally, if after examining the nodule you are uncertain whether it represents an abscess or other inflammatory processes (superficial thrombophlebitis, inflammation of a varicose vein, inflammatory skin nodule), you may want to investigate further by attempting to aspirate the lesion with a needle prior to undertaking a formal incision and drainage procedure. A simple aspiration can help to differentiate between potential abscesses and other conditions that would not be amenable to incision and drainage and may result in harm to patient harm if not identified prior to attempting the procedure.

The following sections will address the typical presentation and evidence-based treatment of abscesses and related conditions. One important note on the treatment of abscesses is the use of post-procedure packing. This was once felt to be tantamount to successful abscess treatment as the belief was held that without packing the wound would heal prematurely necessitating repeat procedures. Numerous randomized controlled trials have investigated the validity of this claim and found that not only does packing not improve outcomes in incision and drainage, but actually prolongs the time to complete healing [63]. Packing also leads to a significant increase in patient pain levels, and many patients do not perform at home dressing changes leading to prolongation of infection [64].

## 9.1  Simple Abscess

Setup for incision and drainage of a simple abscess anywhere on the skin surface should include: syringe and needle for infiltration of anesthetic, anesthetic of choice (I prefer 2 % lidocaine with bicarbonate), iodine, #11 blade, gauze, a bowl of sterile saline, and a hemostat. Gloves must be worn as personal protective equipment; however, they do not need to be sterile gloves nor do you need a sterile field or drape. Abscess incision and drainage is considered a dirty procedure or class IV in the contamination and infection classification of surgical procedures, so sterile technique is not necessary. Draping, however, can be undertaken to protect patient clothing from drainage. In addition you may want to consider wearing mask and goggles as personal protective equipment to prevent accidental splash of infected bodily fluids onto mucosal surfaces. A gown is usually unnecessary but can be utilized at your discretion to protect your clothing from soiling.

Once you have prepped the abscess for incision and drainage, infiltrate the dermis with the anesthetic. Be sure to hold the #11 blade with the blade pointing upward as you carefully enter the skin. The reason for this technique is to prevent from damaging any structures deep to the abscess. The incision should be at least 1.5–2 cm in length to ensure adequate drainage of the cavity. This can be extended to the full length of the abscess if needed. Never make a simple stab incision into an abscess. This can lead to inadequate drainage and clearance of bacteria from the cavity.

Upon entering the cavity, insert a sterile culture swab into the wound to determine the type of bacteria as well as the resistance profile. Be sure to avoid touching the swab to the skin surface, which will contaminate it with skin flora. Determining whether or not the patient has MRSA will help to determine the future of soft tissue infections in this patient.

Once you have drained the purulent material, irrigate the cavity with at least 30 cm³ of sterile saline to remove excessive contamination. After this step, take a piece of stretched out gauze, and using either a hemostat or long cotton swab, push the end into the cavity until the wound is packed. Then slowly remove the gauze. Continue this until you remove any additional gross contamination, usually at least three times. At this point the wound can be left open rather than packed. Packing can lead to prolongation of infection of the wound and prolongation of healing. The wound can be covered with gauze and barrier dressing to prevent soiling of patient clothing.

Antibiotics are unnecessary at this point, as you have removed the source of contamination. Patients can be instructed to shower, wash the wound with soap and water, and change the dressing daily until the wound is fully healed.

## 9.2 Multiloculated Abscess (Carbuncles)

For setup tips and initial procedure, please refer to the preceding section on simple abscess drainage.

When a multiloculated abscess is entered, use a larger incision, at least 3–4 cm in length. After the initial entry is performed with the #11 blade, the loculations can be carefully broken up using a blunt hemostat. Again use care not to enter any structures deep the abscess such as blood vessels. The patient may require additional anesthetic infiltration after the deeper portions of the wound have been entered.

As with simple abscess, upon entering the cavity, insert a sterile culture swab into the wound to determine the type of bacteria as well as the resistance profile. Be sure to avoid touching the swab to the skin surface, which will contaminate it with skin flora. Determining whether or not the patient has MRSA will help to determine the future of soft tissue infections in this patient.

Once you have drained the purulent material, irrigate the cavity with at least 60 mL of sterile saline to remove excessive contamination. After this step, take a piece of stretched out gauze, and using either a hemostat or long cotton swab, push the end into the cavity until the wound is packed. Then slowly remove the gauze. Continue this until you remove any additional gross contamination. At this point the wound can be left open rather than packed. Packing can lead to prolongation of infection of the wound and prolongation of healing. The wound can be covered with gauze and barrier dressing to prevent soiling of patient clothing.

Antibiotics are unnecessary at this point, as you have removed the source of contamination. Patients can be instructed to shower, wash the wound with soap and water, and change the dressing daily until the wound is fully healed.

## 9.3   Paronychia

Paronychia is a type of abscess that occurs along the fold of the nail. There are two types of drainage for paronychia depending on the severity. One is to enter it with an 18 gauge needle and the other is with a #11 blade.

The simplest type of drainage, and the one that should be attempted first, is incision with an 18 gauge needle. This causes the least amount of trauma and discomfort to the patient and can be done without performing a finger block for anesthesia.

**Method 1**

1. Prep the skin and nail with alcohol pad and allow 30 s of drying time. As previously stated, abscess drainage is not a sterile procedure so you can don exam gloves as personal protective equipment. The use of sterile gloves and a sterile field is not necessary.
2. Holding the 18 gauge needle bevel up, slide it along the lateral nail edge entering the space inferior to the nail matrix.
3. Only advance far enough to release the purulent material or until the bevel disappears under the skin.
4. If no purulent material is expressed, then proceed to incision and drainage using a #11 blade.

**Method 2**

1. First prep the finger proximal to the infection with iodine so that you can perform a ring block for anesthesia.
2. Perform the ring block using 2 % lidocaine without epinephrine by inserting the needle into the lateral side of the finger first and advancing until to touch the bone. Retract the needle slightly and infiltrate anesthetic into the area around the nerve. Point the needle toward the palmar surface of the finger and infiltrate anesthetic into this space. Next retract the needle, then redirect toward the dorsum of the finger, and infiltrate anesthetic into this space. Repeat on the medial side of the finger, using between 3 and 5 cm$^3$ of anesthetic, depending on the size of the finger to be anesthetized.
3. Test for adequate anesthesia by touching the tip of the needle to the tip of the finger. If the patient cannot feel the sensation of something sharp, then you are ready to proceed.
4. With the blade pointing toward the nail fold, slide the #11 blade scalpel along the fold and under the nail matrix. This will allow adequate drainage of even small amounts of purulent material that may be trapped under the skin.

After you have finished your procedure, provide an adequate dressing (Band-Aid for a needle drainage or larger gauze dressing for an incision and drainage using a scalpel). Patients should be instructed to soak the wound in 2 cups of water mixed either with 2 tablespoons of Epsom salt or 1 tablespoon of hydrogen peroxide. This can be done for 15 min at least every 4 h for the first 48 h until the wound closes. Antibiotics are unnecessary, unless the cellulitis extends beyond the distal interphalangeal joint.

## 9.4   Infected Sebaceous Cyst

A sebaceous cyst is differentiated from a common abscess in that it is a nodule lined with epithelial cells that contains debris of sloughed cells. It typically presents with a prolonged and indolent course, and the patient may notice that it has been enlarging slowly overtime or that the size has been stable for many months. An infected sebaceous cyst will present as a nodule that suddenly became erythematous, hot, and tender and/or is increasing in size. For complete resolution of a sebaceous cyst, it is necessary to remove the cyst sac, rather than to simply drain the material contained within it. This can be difficult when the cyst becomes infected, however, because the inflammation caused by the infection should be removed in its entirety, without entering the sac, and this will facilitate complete removal. If the sac is entered, it can be removed piecemeal from the wound after drainage.

For this procedure, you will need a #15 blade scalpel, skin hooks or a self-retraction device, blunt forceps (not with teeth), hemostat for blunt dissection, sharp iris scissors for sharp dissection, sterile saline and syringe for irrigation of the cavity, sterile gauze, appropriate suture (5-0 or 4-0 nylon depending on the location), and suture scissors.

1. Prep the skin with iodine. If you are attempting removal of a sebaceous cyst, rather than simple incision and drainage, then full sterile technique should be used (draping and sterile gloves). The reason for this is that, as long as there is no spillage of infected material during the procedure, you can perform skin closure after the removal of the cyst.
2. Carefully infiltrate the skin overlying the cyst with 2 % lidocaine with or without epinephrine for anesthesia. Use caution not to enter or rupture the cyst with the needle while anesthetizing the skin or you will contaminate the procedure.
3. Slowly incise the skin overlying the cyst lengthwise with the #15 blade, using care while advancing the depth of the incision to avoid entering the cyst sac. You will observe the white outer layer of the sac as you incise below the epidermis into the dermis.
4. When you see the cyst sac, place your self-retractor or skin hooks into the epidermis to provide tension between the skin and the sac. This will begin the process of dissection, and you should be able to see the plane of dissection emerging.

5. Using the hemostat and/or iris scissors, dissect around the sac in all directions while holding the cyst gently with the forceps, and then remove it gently from the surrounding tissue.
6. If the cyst is removed intact, you can perform simple interrupted skin closure. If there is any spillage of cyst contents, then leave the wound open.
7. If there is spillage of cyst contents, proceed as with an incision and drainage of abscess. Irrigate the cavity with 30–50 cm$^3$ of sterile saline, and then use the opened piece of gauze to remove gross contamination. If there are portions of the sac visible, you can attempt to remove them in a piecemeal fashion using forceps and iris scissors.

If you were able to close the skin, the sutures can be removed in 7–10 days depending on the tension of the location. If the cyst was not removed, then it should be left open and treated as an abscess. Patients should be informed that there is a high likelihood that the cyst will recur and then can have it removed before it becomes infected.

## 9.5   Infection in the Presence of a Foreign Body

There are many several types of foreign bodies that may be found associated with abscess formation. They can be traumatic, cosmetic, or surgical implants. When an abscess is found to be associated with a foreign body, extensive irrigation should be undertaken to prevent the formation of a fistula at the site. Patients should be informed that the foreign body should be removed as soon as possible. Treating an infected foreign body with antibiotics will only relieve infection temporarily. Antibiotics are not able to clear infection on inorganic materials within the body and will remain as a biofilm covering the object until it is removed.

## 9.6   Necrotizing Infection

It is important to be able to recognize a necrotizing infection presenting to the urgent care so that you can expedite transfer of care to a specialty center with a surgeon on call. Treatment of necrotizing infections is time sensitive, and any patients with signs and symptoms concerning for a necrotizing infection should have an expedited transfer by ambulance to the nearest trauma center.

**Signs and Symptoms**

1. Severe pain out of proportion to physical exam findings
2. Tenderness extending outside the area of erythema
3. Crepitus (presence of trapped gas in the tissues)
4. Signs of systemic toxicity including fever, tachycardia, and/or hypotension
5. Vesicles, bullae, or skin necrosis (later in the course of infection)

Be sure you communicate with the receiving hospital so that they can have a surgical team on standby for when the patient arrives.

## 9.7 Abscesses of Distinct Pathology and Anatomic Location

Many abscesses can be associated with chronic, relapsing disease rather than simple cyst disease or folliculitis. Discretion should be used when treating abscesses relating to these chronic conditions as they tend to recur, and incision and drainage may lead to complications associated with the underlying disease process. Oftentimes, abscesses at these locations can be treated conservatively with appropriate antibiotics and warm compresses or sitz baths. The following sections will address the diagnosis and appropriate treatment of pilonidal disease, Bartholin gland cyst and abscess, and hidradenitis suppurativa.

### 9.7.1 Pilonidal Cyst Disease and Abscess

Pilonidal disease is an inflammatory process that arises from the subcutaneous hair follicles around the intergluteal cleft. It can be recognized by the presence of one or more, small dermal pits. This disease is most common in men from puberty to age 40 and predominantly affects men who sit for prolonged periods of time (truck drivers, office workers, etc.). This disease can be limited to the intergluteal cleft, but chronic disease and abscess may spread to the perianal region and/or anal canal. Patients presenting with pilonidal abscess should have digital rectal examination to rule out deep space infection [65]. As with other soft tissue infections, patients with signs of systemic inflammation (fever, tachycardia, hypotension) should be referred to the Emergency Department for evaluation for potential deep or systemic infection.

Approximately, half of all patients with pilonidal disease will present with an acute abscess at the site of one of the dermal pits [66]. The first episode should be treated with incision and drainage as well as removal of debris and hair follicle (see Sect. 9.1 for technique). The incision should be made laterally along the infected cyst, as midline incisions tend to heal poorly. According to one large study, this procedure results in complete healing of the cyst in one week for about 60 % of cases [67]. However, other more recent studies have reported as high as an 80–90 % recurrence rate for simple incision and drainage alone. Many patients treated in this fashion may go on to develop sinus tracts and chronic relapsing and remitting inflammation. For this reason, it is recommended that patients undergo elliptical excision of the cyst whenever possible with primary closure. One surgical group reported recurrence and chronic disease occurrence as low as 6 % for patients treated in this manner [68].

Patients should be given adequate information about the risk of recurrence and chronic disease at the time of the incision and drainage procedure, so that they know how to seek a consultation from a general surgeon should the disease recur. Hygiene is very important in the prevention of recurrent disease. Patients should be counseled on hair removal from this area and good skin cleansing.

Patients with chronic inflammation of the pilonidal disease, but without abscess, should be referred to a general surgeon for definitive treatment of this disease. Inflammatory disease and cellulitis without abscess should be treated with a 10-day course of antibiotics, typically 500 mg of ciprofloxacin twice daily combined with 500 mg of metronidazole three times daily. The patient should be instructed on performing sitz baths (15 min in a tub with 1 cup of Epsom salt dissolved in warm water) to encourage the drainage of sinus tracts and improve inflammation.

| Acute abscess | Chronic disease with cellulitis |
| --- | --- |
| • Incision and drainage (lateral to the abscess) | • Antibiotics (fluoroquinolone + metronidazole) |
| • Sitz baths | • Sitz baths |
| • Good hygiene | • General surgery referral |
| • Counseling on recurrence | |

## 9.7.2  Bartholin Gland Cyst and Abscess

Bartholin glands are typically small, non-palpable, mucous-secreting organs located bilaterally near the posterior opening of the vagina. Obstruction of the duct can lead the glands to fill with mucous, resulting in Bartholin gland cysts. Predisposing factors to the formation of a cyst are local trauma, infection (such as sexually transmitted infections (STI)), stenosis of the duct, or tumor. It is especially common in younger women, and incidence typically decreases with age. All women should be counseled on the risk of an associated STI and undergo appropriate testing for gonorrhea and chlamydia. In addition women over 40 who present with Bartholin gland cyst or abscess have a higher risk of associated cancer and should be immediately referred to a specialist for removal and biopsy. Asymptomatic cysts rarely require treatment [69].

When the cyst becomes infected with bacteria, it can quickly develop into an abscess. Signs of abscess include pain and swelling of the labia majora, pain with walking, and/or pain with intercourse.

Treatment for Bartholin gland abscess can be staged due to severity on presentation, as incision and drainage of these abscesses is an inferior procedure to either Word catheter placement [70] or marsupialization [71]. Incision and drainage alone can also make later definitive treatment difficult. If you are near an Emergency Department capable of performing either placement of a Word catheter or marsupialization, then patients should be triaged to the ED for appropriate management. Abscesses of Bartholin gland cysts tend to recur if not treated appropriately, and repeated incision and drainage needs to be avoided if possible.

If you do not have access to an Emergency Department and are unfamiliar with either marsupialization or Word catheter placement, then the following treatment algorithm can be employed:

1. Conservative Management: Advise patient on the use of sitz baths (15 min of soaking in a bathtub of warm water combined with 1 cup Epsom salt) 3–4 times daily to encourage spontaneous drainage. These patients should also be treated with broad-spectrum antibiotic (cephalexin 500 mg four times daily for 7–10 days) to lessen the degree of associated cellulitis of the labia majora.
2. Incision and Drainage: For patients with very large, painful abscesses or who have failed at least 3 days of conservative management, standard incision and drainage can be undertaken in the urgent care setting (see Sect. 9.1 for instructions). This procedure can alleviate pain and prevent further complications, although it is not the preferred method of treatment as discussed above. Note that the incision should not be made through the skin of the labia majora; rather, the abscess should be incised vertically, near the location of the normal Bartholin gland opening, through the mucocutaneous junction on the posterior lateral wall of the vaginal introitus. After the cysts has been evacuated and irrigated, application of silver nitrate to the cyst cavity has shown a decrease in recurrence rate [72]. After incision and drainage, antibiotics should be continued for the full 7–10-day course.

Patients need to be counseled that without definitive treatment by an experienced gynecologist, the cyst will likely recur. Definitive treatment entails either placement of a Word catheter or marsupialization and is beyond the scope of this book.

**Treatment Algorithm of Bartholin Gland Abscess**
- Antibiotics alone for small, minimally painful abscess with referral to gynecology
- Testing for sexually transmitted infections (STI)
- Large, painful abscess—triage to provider capable of performing Word catheter insertion or marsupialization
- Incision and drainage with silver nitrate application as a last resort

## 9.7.3   Hidradenitis Suppurativa

Hidradenitis suppurativa (HS) is a chronic disease that results from inflammation of the apocrine glands in the groin, axilla, inframammary, perineal, and perianal regions [73]. This disease results in chronic infections, abscesses, sinus tracts, and draining wounds that can become debilitating and painful. Evaluation of the skin may reveal comedones or pits in the skin, ropelike contractures and/or sinus tracts, erythematous nodules and/or papules, and/or tender abscesses and draining papules. Patient history concerning for hidradenitis includes: presence of active disease and history of three or more discharging nodules or abscesses in the same location since the age of 10 or history of 5 or more discharging lesions or abscesses in the same location since the age of 10 without active disease. The most commonly used system for identifying and classifying HS is the Hurley staging system [74]. Stage 1 of HS is characterized by recurrent abscesses without sinus tract formation, stage 2 by one or more sinus tracts separated by normal skin, and stage 3 by multiple connected sinus tracts without normal skin.

It is important to recognize HS in patients presenting with an abscess in one of these locations as repeated incision and drainage can result in increased formation of sinus tracts and worsening of the chronic inflammation associated with this disease. Repeated attempts and incision and drainage can also accelerate scarring, keloid formation, and contractures associated with this disease.

1. Conservative Management: Localized disease can be treated with warm compresses and antibiotics such as doxycycline, minocycline, trimethoprim sulfamethoxazole, clindamycin, or dapsone.
2. Incision and Drainage: If there is an abscess present that is causing severe pain and cellulitis, then incision and drainage may be undertaken to relieve the patient's symptoms. This can be performed in the same method as for simple abscess drainage. All patients should be continued on antibiotics for at least a 7–10-day course to prevent relapse of the disease during healing.

Patients with potential diagnosis of hidradenitis suppurativa can be referred back to their primary care physician for localized treatment of the disease, especially if this is the first time that an abscess has developed at the site. Patients should not be continued on oral antibiotic monotherapy long term due to the risk of developing resistance in the infecting organisms. Other treatments can include antibacterial wash, topical clindamycin, topical retinoids, hormonal therapies, systemic retinoids, and intralesional steroid injections [75]. Most of these treatments are only temporarily effective against this disease, and providers have been turning to alternatives including immunomodulatory therapy [76, 77]. Patients with recurrent abscesses, sinus tracts, contractures, widely separated lesions, or diffuse disease should be referred to general surgery for wide local excision and primary closure [78].

# Chapter 10
# Burns

The following section contains the most current consensus and evidence-based recommendations for burn treatment. These guidelines are endorsed by the American Burn Association and are based on two large reviews entitled Practice Guidelines for Burn Care [79].

Many patients will present to the urgent care with burns. The most important part of treating burns in the urgent care is first to determine the degree and extent of the burn.

All burn patients are first of all trauma patients. They should be assessed for other life-threatening injuries prior to assessment of the burn. All assessments should begin with ABCs (airway, breathing, and circulation). It is imperative that all patients with burns have an airway assessment first and foremost. Patients with inhalation injury can rapidly decompensate and early endotracheal intubation is necessary. If the patient presents with burns while in an enclosed space, flash burns to the face, singed nose hairs, erythema of the mouth and pharynx, hoarse voice, wheezing, or dyspnea [80], call 911.

Once you have completed the primary assessment, then move on to the burn-specific assessment.

## 10.1   Classifying a Burn

First-Degree Burns: Burn limited to the epidermis (most common type is a sunburn). The burned site is red and painful; there are no blisters. This type of burn requires limited intervention and will heal without any long-term complications.

Second-Degree Burns: Two types of burns fall into this category, superficial burns to the papillary dermis and deep burns to the reticular dermis. Superficial second-degree burns are characterized by blanching erythema, blistering, and pain. Deep second-degree burns lead to injury of the nerves and result in decreased sensation and blistering with a loss of hair follicles. Deep second-degree burns will require excision and skin grafting and should be referred to a burn treatment center.

© Springer International Publishing Switzerland 2016
B. Busse, *Wound Management in Urgent Care*,
DOI 10.1007/978-3-319-27428-7_10

Third-Degree Burns: This is a burn that penetrates the dermis and results in damage to the subcutaneous fat. These burns are often white, dry or charred, leathery feeling, and painless. Third-degree burns warrant immediate transfer to a burn treatment center.

Fourth-Degree Burns: These burns penetrate to bone, muscle, and tendon. They will also be white and/or charred and painless. Again, these burns require immediate transfer to a burn treatment center.

## 10.2   Assessment of Burn Surface Area (BSA)

The easiest way to assess the surface area of a burn is to use Wallace's "rule of nines." Be aware that only second-degree burns and deeper will be included in the estimation. First-degree burns can be easily treated in the home with supportive care no matter the extent.

Wallace's Rule of Nines

- Head = 9, arms = 9 each, chest = 18, back = 18, legs = 18 each, perineum = 1

You can also use the patient's palm as an estimation tool; 1 palm = 0.5 % TBSA burn [81]. This has been found to be the most accurate method for estimating burn size, especially for irregular burns. (This is different than previously held belief that one palm = 1 % TBSA).

## 10.3   Burn Center Admission Criteria

Establishing a relationship with the nearest burn specialty treatment center or with the nearest local Emergency Department if you are not located within 50 miles of a burn center is critical to caring for burns in the urgent care setting. If patients are unstable and require intubation or fluid resuscitation, they should be transported by ambulance to the nearest Emergency Department. For stable patients, the burn specialty center can often be contacted directly for patients meeting admission criteria or for those patients who will require follow-up for wound care and monitoring.

The following are the most current admission criteria for hospitals and burn specialty centers [82]:

- Second- and third-degree burns >10 % BSA in patients age <10 or >50
- Second- and third-degree burns >20 % BSA in all other patients
- Second- and third-degree burns to the hands, feet, face, genitals, perineum, or skin overlying major joints
- Third-degree burns >5 % BSA in all patients
- Electrical or chemical burns
- Concomitant trauma, inhalation injury, or preexisting medical conditions that may impair healing

- Burns in patients requiring social and/or emotional support, or long-term rehabilitation
- Suspected abuse or neglect
  - Important points:

    Delayed presentation
    Conflicting history
    Previous injures

  - Physical exam findings:

    Sharply demarcated
    Uniform depth
    Absence of splash marks
    Stocking or glove pattern
    Flexor sparing
    Dorsal location on the hands
    Very deep localized contact

**Risk Factors for Inhalation Injury**
- Alcohol use
- Trauma
- Enclosed space
- Rapid combustion
- Extremely young or old
- Prolonged extrication

## 10.4   Caring for Burns in the Urgent Care

Once you have determined that the burn does not require hospital admission, fluid resuscitation, or referral to a burn specialty center, you can treat the burn in the urgent care.

1. Provide the patient with adequate pain control. Ensure that they have a ride home. If they are alone and do not have anyone to come to assist them, then they should be transferred to a hospital for inpatient care due to need to social support.
2. Burns should be carefully washed and debrided. This may include removing dirt and debris from deep friction burn as well as necrotic skin from ruptured blisters. Several studies have investigated whether or not intact blisters should be drained or ruptured. These studies found that blisters should be left intact if possible as it improves healing and decreases burn infection [83].
3. Cooling on the burn wound has only been shown to be effective when started in the first two minutes after injury and should be continued for only 20–30 min. Do not apply ice to the skin. Rather, apply cool towels to the skin or bathe in cool water.

4. A thin layer of moisture-retentive ointment should be applied to all burned surfaces. Antibacterial ointment such as bacitracin or neosporin can be used if that is all you have available; however, it is preferable to use a petroleum-based ointment like Aquaphor or aloe-containing ointments to prevent superinfection of wounds with pseudomonas [84].

   (a) Silvadene (silver sulfadiazine): Although this was once seen as preferential in outpatient burn wound treatment, its use has been limited in the care of burns among burn specialists. This topical antimicrobial cream has many drawbacks including pain with application, limited eschar penetration, and potential to cause neutropenia and thrombocytopenia. This topical antimicrobial should be limited to use in infected burns and cannot be used in patients with an allergy to Sulfa medications.

5. A nonadherent Telfa dressing should be used to cover the wounds, and then the wounds can be wrapped with gauze dressing. Do not apply gauze directly to the burn wounds as it will stick and result in significant patient discomfort when removed.

6. Netted stockings can be placed over the gauze to keep the dressing in place and can be reused by patients for at-home dressing changes.

7. Patients should be instructed to premedicate with analgesics before changing the dressing (and given adequate analgesics to do so, as well as dressing materials). This should be done on a daily basis, and wounds will need to be adequately washed and patted dry to prevent bacterial infection. Patients need to have any adequate support system at home to assist with dressing changes. Patients who do not have adequate home support would qualify for inpatient admission to a hospital and/or burn specialty center.

8. Patients should be referred back to their primary care physician or to the local burn specialty center, if available, for weekly or biweekly evaluations and dressing changes.

There is no role for prophylactic antibiotics in the treatment of burn wounds.

All patients should receive tetanus toxoid immunization if their tetanus vaccination is inadequate or unknown.

With adequate evaluation and early intervention with proper referral, the urgent care provider can treat most burn wounds successfully.

# Chapter 11
# Chronic Wounds

There are many conditions that can lead to chronic open wounds that may be evaluated in the urgent care setting. Patients with diabetes, peripheral vascular disease, venous stasis, congestive heart failure, lymphedema, and/or impaired mobility are all at risk for developing wounds that are difficult to heal. Categorization of the type and cause of a wound is important for diagnosis in that the underlying disease process will need to be appropriately managed, typically by the primary care physician. The most important aspects of wound care management in the urgent care will be to initiate wound dressings and to identify any potential infection. Patients may also present with traumatic or postsurgical wounds requesting an evaluation or dressing change. The same principles of wound treatment will be applied with referral to the surgeon after treatment has been initiated.

The following will outline the basics of caring for open wounds, followed by sections that will provide a brief overview of several types of wounds that may present to the urgent care for treatment, as well as any points that should be addressed in each specialized case.

## 11.1  Basics of Initial Evaluation and Treatment of Chronic Wounds

No matter the cause of the wound, when dealing with wounds in the urgent care, your focus will be on removing devitalized tissue and debris, reducing bacterial load, identifying and treating soft tissue infection, and initiating the process of wound healing by secondary intention. Following the initial treatment, ensure that patients receive appropriate referrals either directly to a wound care specialist if you are able or back to their primary care physician.

© Springer International Publishing Switzerland 2016
B. Busse, *Wound Management in Urgent Care*,
DOI 10.1007/978-3-319-27428-7_11

1. After donning sterile personal protective equipment, including gown, sterile gloves, and eye protection, prep the surrounding skin with either chlorhexidine or povidone-iodine solution, and prepare a sterile field to lessen bacterial contamination of the wound during the procedure.
2. Infiltrate a local anesthetic into the skin and tissues surrounding the wound, including the base of the wound. For large wounds it is better to use 1 % lidocaine rather than 2 % to lower the risk of overdose and systemic toxicity.
3. All nonviable or necrotic material needs to be debrided from the wound. This can be accomplished using a #10 blade scalpel, forceps, and iris scissors. Eschar needs to be carefully trimmed away from the edges and base of the wound. Any questionably viable tissue can be left on the wound to be removed later during dressing changes.
4. Following debridement, the wound should be irrigated under low pressure with normal saline to lessen bacterial contamination. Harsh antimicrobials like iodine, hydrogen peroxide, and chlorhexidine should not be used as they can lead to desiccation of tissue and further tissue necrosis. Low-pressure irrigation can be performed using a saline bag in a pressure cuff (a sphygmomanometer can be used if you have nothing else available) hooked up to I.V. tubing and a 19 gauge angiocatheter.
5. Wet-to-dry dressings can be used in most initial situations. They are an optimal initial wound dressing, as they are easy to administer, have low initial cost, and provide a moist environment that encourages secondary wound healing and formation of granulation tissue, and their removal results in debridement of the wound of exudate and superficial tissue [85]. Patients and patient care representatives should be instructed on the dressing of the wound so that it can be changed twice daily. They should be given adequate materials to perform dressing changes until follow-up with the primary care physician or specialist can be arranged. Many nursing professionals have argued for the use of alginate or foam dressings which have shown evidence of decreased patient discomfort and nursing costs [86]; however, surgical research has shown no superiority for these types of dressings over standard gauze wet-to-dry dressings in terms of time to full healing, and the material cost is significantly less than for occlusive dressings [87]. Negative pressure wound therapy has been advocated to treat many types of lower extremity and pressure ulcers. At this time there is no good evidence to support its use over topical dressing changes [88, 89]. Patients should have an evaluation by a wound care specialist in a reasonable amount of time for continued dressing changes or evaluation for negative pressure wound therapy.
6. Signs of wound infection include malodorous discharge, surrounding erythema, edema, warmth, and/or tenderness to palpation. Cellulitis should be treated using an antibiotic effective against *Staphylococcus* and *Streptococcus* species such as cephalexin 500 mg orally four times per day. Infected diabetic foot ulcers or pressure ulcers typically contain gram-negative bacteria, and therefore, clindamycin 300 mg orally three times daily or trimethoprim-sulfamethoxazole DS twice daily may be added. Many patients with chronic wounds may be at risk

for MRSA infection, so TMP-sulfa, clindamycin, or levofloxacin could be added to most treatment regimens.

## 11.2   Special Types of Wounds

### 11.2.1   Diabetic Foot Ulcers

Diabetic patients are prone to developing ulcerations of the feet due to neuropathy and possible concomitant arterial occlusive disease leading to poor wound healing. In any diabetic patient presenting with leg edema and possible cellulitis, a thorough inspection of the foot should be undertaken for wounds, especially between the toes in the webspace and along the nail edge. An adequate history of the ulcer should be obtained and should include length of time the ulcer has been present, history of mechanical trauma or poorly fitting shoes, as well as previous treatment to this ulcer. In addition, obtain a history of similar ulcer, whether or not they healed spontaneously, and over what length of time. Finally, the initial evaluation should include history of recent blood sugar testing, as uncontrolled hyperglycemia may be the only indication of infection in a diabetic patient with impaired sensation and arterial blood flow.

Diabetic patients may present with deep ulcerations, severe cellulitis, and/or necrotizing infections due to loss of sensation of the foot. An X-ray should be obtained before initiating any treatment to rule out the presence of gangrene or osteomyelitis. Either of these conditions would necessitate transfer to a local emergency room with on-call surgical capabilities for orthopedic and/or vascular surgery.

### 11.2.2   Arterial Occlusive Disease

Patients with peripheral arterial occlusive disease may present to the urgent care with nonhealing wounds of the lower extremity or dry gangrene. It is important to obtain history of risk factors including cigarette smoking, hyperlipidemia, and diabetes mellitus. Also patients should be questioned about prior surgical history, especially relating to lower extremity revascularization procedures, catheterizations, coronary artery bypass, and carotid endarterectomy.

Physical examination should include palpation of distal pulses including those of the dorsalis pedis, posterior tibial, popliteal, and femoral arteries bilaterally. Patients with suspected arterial occlusive disease should be referred back to the primary care physician or to a vascular surgeon for further diagnostic testing and follow-up after initiation of wound treatment. Patients with critical limb ischemia and signs of infection should be transferred to a local Emergency Department with on-call vascular surgery consultation available.

## 11.2.3   Venous Insufficiency

Venous insufficiency can be a result of severe chronic varicose veins or following deep venous thrombosis. The skin will demonstrate loss of hair distally and/or hyperpigmentation from deposition of hemosiderin. The skin will begin to lose subcutaneous fat and become thin and leathery. Ulcerations often develop, particularly on the medial side. These ulcerations are shallow, typically bleed easily due to the presence of granulation tissue, and may be covered with fibrinous yellow exudate. The ulcer and surrounding skin should be evaluated for signs of infection. This can be tricky as the lower limb of a patient with venous insufficiency may be chronically edematous, and the patient may develop erythema and dilation of the capillaries consistent with dependent rubor. Dependent rubor can be distinguished from the erythema and edema associated with infection by having the patient lie supine on the bed and elevating the lower extremity. The skin should slowly begin to blanch with elevation in the case of dependent rubor, but not with infection. Malodorous discharge from the wound is also a sign of infection.

## 11.2.4   Decubitus (Pressure) Ulcers

The National Pressure Ulcer Advisory Panel (NPUAP) defines a pressure ulcer as an area of unrelieved pressure, typically over a boney prominence, that results in tissue ischemia, cell death, and tissue necrosis. They are typically seen in persons who are incapacitated due to physical or mental illness and especially those persons who are reliant on others for changes in positioning.

Pressure ulcers should be staged according to NPUAP guidelines as follows [90]:

1. Suspected: Deep purple or maroon discoloration of the skin or blood-filled blister due to damage of the underlying tissue from pressure or shear
2. Stage I: Signs of impending ulceration including blanchable erythema and reactive hyperemia
3. Stage II: A partial thickness loss of skin including the epidermis and dermis
4. Stage III: A full thickness loss of skin with extension into underlying soft tissue that does not violate the fascia
5. Stage IV: A full thickness loss of skin and underlying tissue including muscle, bone, and tendon or with extension into the joint capsule
6. Unstageable: A full thickness tissue loss where the base is covered by slough or eschar so that the full extent of penetration is not immediately apparent

Successful treatment of pressure ulcers is reliant on adequate staging (debridement and eschar removal if present), relief of pressure, control of infection, and local wound care.

Epidermis

Dermis

Subcutaneous Fat

Soft Tissue

Bone

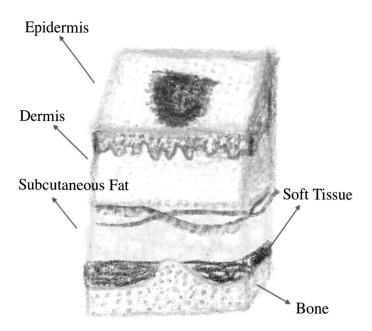

Stage I decubitus ulcer

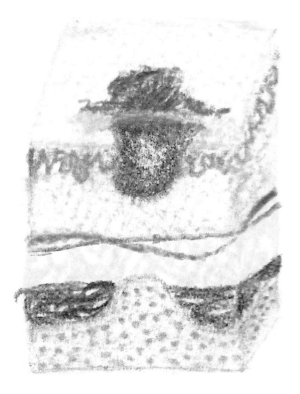

Stage II decubitus ulcer

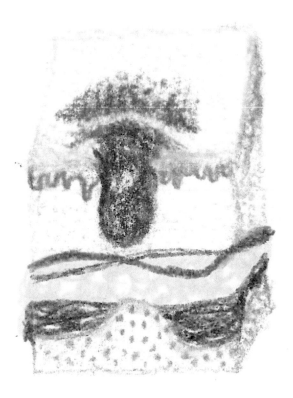

Stage III decubitus ulcer

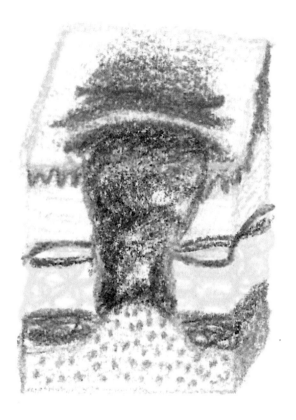

Stage IV decubitus ulcer

# References

1. Bertone AL. Principles of wound healing. Vet Clin North Am Equine Pract. 1989;5(3):449–63.
2. Hackam DJ, Ford HR. Cellular, biochemical, and clinical aspects of wound healing. Surg Infect (Larchmt). 2002;3 Suppl 1:S23–35.
3. Singer AJ, Clark RA. Cutaneous wound healing. N Engl J Med. 1999;341(10):738–46.
4. Yamaguchi Y, Yoshikawa K. Cutaneous wound healing: an update. J Dermatol. 2001;28(10):521–34.
5. Heldin CH, Ostman A, Westermark B. Structure of platelet-derived growth factor: implications for functional properties. Growth Factors. 1993;8(4):245–52.
6. Braiman-Wiksman L, Solomonik I, Spira R, Tennenbaum T. Novel insights into wound healing sequence of events. Toxicol Pathol. 2007;35(6):767–79.
7. Rodero MP, Khosrotehrani K. Skin wound healing modulation by macrophages. Int J Clin Exp Pathol. 2010;3(7):643–53.
8. Leibovich SJ, Ross R. The role of the macrophage in wound repair. A study with hydrocortisone and antimacrophage serum. Am J Pathol. 1975;78(1):71–100.
9. Mirza R, DiPietro LA, Koh TJ. Selective and specific macrophage ablation is detrimental to wound healing in mice. Am J Pathol. 2009;175(6):2454–62.
10. Greiling D, Clark RA. Fibronectin provides a conduit for fibroblast transmigration from collagenous stroma into fibrin clot provisional matrix. J Cell Sci. 1997;110(Pt 7):861–70.
11. Sidgwick GP, McGeorge D, Bayat A. A comprehensive evidence-based review on the role of topicals and dressings in the management of skin scarring. Arch Dermatol Res. 2015;307(6):461–77.
12. Chatterjee JS. A critical review of irrigation techniques in acute wounds. Int Wound J. 2005;2(3):258–65.
13. van den Baar MT, van der Palen J, Vroon MI, Bertelink P, Hendrix R. Is time to closure a factor in the occurrence of infection in traumatic wounds? A prospective cohort study in a Dutch level 1 trauma centre. Emerg Med J. 2010;27(7):540–3.
14. Dire DJ, Coppola M, Dwyer DA, Lorette JJ, Karr JL. Prospective evaluation of topical antibiotics for preventing infections in uncomplicated soft-tissue wounds repaired in the ED. Acad Emerg Med. 1995;2(1):4–10.
15. Holt DR, Kirk SJ, Regan MC, Hurson M, Lindblad WJ, Barbul A. Effect of age on wound healing in healthy human beings. Surgery. 1992;112(2):293–7; discussion 297–8.
16. Hopf HW, Hunt TK, West JM, et al. Wound tissue oxygen tension predicts the risk of wound infection in surgical patients. Arch Surg. 1997;132(9):997–1004; discussion 1005.
17. Mosely LH, Finseth F, Goody M. Nicotine and its effect on wound healing. Plast Reconstr Surg. 1978;61(4):570–5.

18. Goodson 3rd WH, Hung TK. Studies of wound healing in experimental diabetes mellitus. J Surg Res. 1977;22(3):221–7.
19. Williams JZ, Barbul A. Nutrition and wound healing. Surg Clin North Am. 2003;83(3):571–96.
20. Hunt TK. Vitamin A, and wound healing. J Am Acad Dermatol. 1986;15(4 Pt 2):817–21.
21. Anstead GM. Steroids, retinoids, and wound healing. Adv Wound Care. 1998;11(6):277–85.
22. Saper RB, Rash R. Zinc: an essential micronutrient. Am Fam Physician. 2009;79(9):768–72.
23. Postlethwait RW. Long-term comparative study of nonabsorbable sutures. Ann Surg. 1970;171(6):892–8.
24. Fomete B, Saheeb BD, Obiadazie AC. A prospective clinical evaluation of the longevity of resorbable sutures in oral surgical procedures. Niger J Clin Pract. 2013;16(3):334–8.
25. Tejani C, Sivitz AB, Rosen MD, et al. A comparison of cosmetic outcomes of lacerations on the extremities and trunk using absorbable versus nonabsorbable sutures. Acad Emerg Med. 2014;21(6):637–43.
26. Abidin MR, Becker DG, Paley RD, et al. A new compound curved needle for intradermal suture closure. J Emerg Med. 1989;7(5):441–4.
27. Farion K, Osmond MH, Hartling L, et al. Tissue adhesives for traumatic lacerations in children and adults. Cochrane Database Syst Rev. 2002;3, CD003326.
28. Baker MD, Lanuti M. The management and outcome of lacerations in urban children. Ann Emerg Med. 1990;19(9):1001–5.
29. Kanegaye JT, Vance CW, Chan L, Schonfeld N. Comparison of skin stapling devices and standard sutures for pediatric scalp lacerations: a randomized study of cost and time benefits. J Pediatr. 1997;130(5):808–13.
30. Hollander JE, Richman PB, Werblud M, Miller T, Huggler J, Singer AJ. Irrigation in facial and scalp lacerations: does it alter outcome? Ann Emerg Med. 1998;31(1):73–7.
31. Hock MO, Ooi SB, Saw SM, Lim SH. A randomized controlled trial comparing the hair apposition technique with tissue glue to standard suturing in scalp lacerations (HAT study). Ann Emerg Med. 2002;40(1):19–26.
32. Ozturk D, Sonmez BM, Altinbilek E, Kavalci C, Arslan ED, Akay S. A retrospective observational study comparing hair apposition technique, suturing and stapling for scalp lacerations. World J Emerg Surg. 2013;8:27.
33. Park SW, Oh TS, Choi JW, et al. Topical EMLA cream as a pretreatment for facial lacerations. Arch Plast Surg. 2015;42(1):28–33.
34. Evans R, Jones J. Best evidence topic report. Absorbable sutures in paediatric lacerations. Emerg Med J. 2006;23(1):64–5.
35. Beam JW. Tissue adhesives for simple traumatic lacerations. J Athl Train. 2008;43(2):222–4.
36. Smith J, Maconochie I. Should we glue lip lacerations in children? Arch Dis Child. 2003;88(1):83–4.
37. Smith TO, Sexton D, Mann C, Donell S. Sutures versus staples for skin closure in orthopaedic surgery: meta-analysis. BMJ. 2010;340:c1199.
38. Payne RL, Martin ML. Defining and classifying skin tears: need for a common language. Ostomy Wound Manage. 1993;39(5):16–20; 22–14, 26.
39. LeBlanc K, Baranoski S, Skin Tear Consensus Panel Members. Skin tears: state of the science: consensus statements for the prevention, prediction, assessment, and treatment of skin tears©. Adv Skin Wound Care. 2011;24(9 Suppl):2–15.
40. Baranoski S. How to prevent and manage skin tears. Adv Skin Wound Care. 2003;16(5):268–70.
41. Leblanc K, Baranoski S. Prevention and management of skin tears. Adv Skin Wound Care. 2009;22(7):325–32; quiz 333–4.
42. Bank D, Nix D. Preventing skin tears in a nursing and rehabilitation center: an interdisciplinary effort. Ostomy Wound Manage. 2006;52(9):38–40; 44, 46.
43. White MW, Karam S, Cowell B. Skin tears in frail elders: a practical approach to prevention. Geriatr Nurs. 1994;15(2):95–9.

44. Carville K, Lewin G, Newall N, et al. STAR: a consensus for skin tear classification. Primary Intention. 2007;15(1):18–28.

45. Ayello EA, Sibbald RG. A new global perspective of evidence-based wound protocols. Adv Skin Wound Care. 2006;19(8):416–9.

46. Fleck CA. Preventing and treating skin tears. Adv Skin Wound Care. 2007;20(6):315–20.

47. Milne CT, Corbett LQ. A new option in the treatment of skin tears for the institutionalized resident: formulated 2-octylcyanoacrylate topical bandage. Geriatr Nurs. 2005;26(5):321–5.

48. Edwards H, Gaskill D, Nash R. Treating skin tears in nursing home residents: a pilot study comparing four types of dressings. Int J Nurs Pract. 1998;4(1):25–32.

49. Lackmann GM, Draf W, Isselstein G, Tollner U. Surgical treatment of facial dog bite injuries in children. J Craniomaxillofac Surg. 1992;20(2):81–6.

50. Rui-feng C, Li-song H, Ji-bo Z, Li-qiu W. Emergency treatment on facial laceration of dog bite wounds with immediate primary closure: a prospective randomized trial study. BMC Emerg Med. 2013;13 Suppl 1:S2.

51. Cheng HT, Hsu YC, Wu CI. Does primary closure for dog bite wounds increase the incidence of wound infection? A meta-analysis of randomized controlled trials. J Plast Reconstr Aesthet Surg. 2014;67(10):1448–50.

52. Medeiros I, Saconato H. Antibiotic prophylaxis for mammalian bites. Cochrane Database Syst Rev. 2001;2, CD001738.

53. Esposito S, Picciolli I, Semino M, Principi N. Dog and cat bite-associated infections in children. Eur J Clin Microbiol Infect Dis. 2013;32(8):971–6.

54. Brook I. Management of human and animal bite wound infection: an overview. Curr Infect Dis Rep. 2009;11(5):389–95.

55. Rothe K, Tsokos M, Handrick W. Animal and human bite wounds. Dtsch Arztebl Int. 2015;112(25):433–42; quiz 443.

56. Myers JP. Bite wound infections. Curr Infect Dis Rep. 2003;5(5):416–25.

57. Cook CP, Knox MJ, Wimberly RL, Ellis HB, Riccio AI. "Fight-bite": not just a hand problem. J Pediatr Orthop. 2014;34(6):647–9.

58. Donkor P, Bankas DO. A study of primary closure of human bite injuries to the face. J Oral Maxillofac Surg. 1997;55(5):479–81; discussion 481–2.

59. Patil PD, Panchabhai TS, Galwankar SC. Managing human bites. J Emerg Trauma Shock. 2009;2(3):186–90.

60. Conlon HA. Human bites in the classroom: incidence, treatment, and complications. J Sch Nurs. 2007;23(4):197–201.

61. Cooper KL. Evidence-based prevention of pressure ulcers in the intensive care unit. Crit Care Nurse. 2013;33(6):57–66.

62. Fahimi J, Singh A, Frazee BW. The role of adjunctive antibiotics in the treatment of skin and soft tissue abscesses: a systematic review and meta-analysis. CJEM. 2015;17(4):420–32.

63. Kessler DO, Krantz A, Mojica M. Randomized trial comparing wound packing to no wound packing following incision and drainage of superficial skin abscesses in the pediatric emergency department. Pediatr Emerg Care. 2012;28(6):514–7.

64. O'Malley GF, Dominici P, Giraldo P, et al. Routine packing of simple cutaneous abscesses is painful and probably unnecessary. Acad Emerg Med. 2009;16(5):470–3.

65. Vallance S. Pilonidal fistulas mimicking fistulas-in-ano. Br J Surg. 1982;69(3):161–2.

66. Allen-Mersh TG. Pilonidal sinus: finding the right track for treatment. Br J Surg. 1990;77(2):123–32.

67. Lord PH, Millar DM. Pilonidal sinus: a simple treatment. Br J Surg. 1965;52:298–300.

68. Ciftci F, Abdurrahman I, Tosun M, Bas G. A new approach: oblique excision and primary closure in the management of acute pilonidal disease. Int J Clin Exp Med. 2014;7(12):5706–10.

69. Hill DA, Lense JJ. Office management of Bartholin gland cysts and abscesses. Am Fam Physician. 1998;57(7):1611–6; 1619–20.

70. Word B. Office treatment of cyst and abscess of Bartholin's gland duct. South Med J. 1968;61(5):514–8.

71. Mathews D. Marsupialization in the treatment of Bartholin's cysts and abscesses. J Obstet Gynaecol Br Commonw. 1966;73(6):1010–2.
72. Wechter ME, Wu JM, Marzano D, Haefner H. Management of Bartholin duct cysts and abscesses: a systematic review. Obstet Gynecol Surv. 2009;64(6):395–404.
73. Jansen I, Altmeyer P, Piewig G. Acne inversa (alias hidradenitis suppurativa). J Eur Acad Dermatol Venereol. 2001;15(6):532–40.
74. Gill L, Williams M, Hamzavi I. Update on hidradenitis suppurativa: connecting the tracts. F1000Prime Rep. 2014;6:112.
75. Rambhatla PV, Lim HW, Hamzavi I. A systematic review of treatments for hidradenitis suppurativa. Arch Dermatol. 2012;148(4):439–46.
76. Moriarty B, Jiyad Z, Creamer D. Four-weekly infliximab in the treatment of severe hidradenitis suppurativa. Br J Dermatol. 2014;170(4):986–7.
77. Kimball AB, Kerdel F, Adams D, et al. Adalimumab for the treatment of moderate to severe Hidradenitis suppurativa: a parallel randomized trial. Ann Intern Med. 2012;157(12):846–55.
78. Blok JL, Spoo JR, Leeman FW, Jonkman MF, Horvath B. Skin-tissue-sparing excision with electrosurgical peeling (STEEP): a surgical treatment option for severe hidradenitis suppurativa Hurley stage II/III. J Eur Acad Dermatol Venereol. 2015;29(2):379–82.
79. Gibran NS, Committee on Organization and Delivery of Burn Care, American Burn Association. Practice guidelines for burn care, 2006. J Burn Care Res. 2006;27(4):437–8.
80. Tredget EE, Shankowsky HA, Taerum TV, Moysa GL, Alton JD. The role of inhalation injury in burn trauma. A Canadian experience. Ann Surg. 1990;212(6):720–7.
81. Sheridan RL, Petras L, Basha G, et al. Planimetry study of the percent of body surface represented by the hand and palm: sizing irregular burns is more accurately done with the palm. J Burn Care Rehabil. 1995;16(6):605–6.
82. Guidelines for the operation of burn centers. American burn association and American college of surgeons. Bull Am Coll Surg. 1995;80(10):34–41.
83. Swain AH, Azadian BS, Wakeley CJ, Shakespeare PG. Management of blisters in minor burns. Br Med J (Clin Res Ed). 1987;295(6591):181.
84. Heinrich JJ, Brand DA, Cuono CB. The role of topical treatment as a determinant of infection in outpatient burns. J Burn Care Rehabil. 1988;9(3):253–7.
85. Vermeulen H, Ubbink D, Goossens A, de Vos R, Legemate D. Dressings and topical agents for surgical wounds healing by secondary intention. Cochrane Database Syst Rev. 2004;2, CD003554.
86. Ovington LG. Hanging wet-to-dry dressings out to dry. Home Healthc Nurse. 2001;19(8):477–83; quiz 484.
87. Ubbink DT, Vermeulen H, Goossens A, Kelner RB, Schreuder SM, Lubbers MJ. Occlusive vs gauze dressings for local wound care in surgical patients: a randomized clinical trial. Arch Surg. 2008;143(10):950–5.
88. Dumville JC, Land L, Evans D, Peinemann F. Negative pressure wound therapy for treating leg ulcers. Cochrane Database Syst Rev. 2015;7, CD011354.
89. Dumville JC, Webster J, Evans D, Land L. Negative pressure wound therapy for treating pressure ulcers. Cochrane Database Syst Rev. 2015;5, CD011334.
90. Stausberg J, Kiefer E. Classification of pressure ulcers: a systematic literature review. Stud Health Technol Inform. 2009;146:511–5.

# Index

## A
Abscess, 61–70
Absorbable sutures, 19, 20
Adhesive strip, 9, 19, 22, 23, 60
Aftercare, 3, 61
Animal bite
   cat, 57, 58
   dog, 57, 58
   human, 57–59
Arterial disease, 77
Avulsion, 53

## B
Bacitracin, 8, 31, 33, 36, 38, 39, 41, 43, 45,
     47, 49, 51, 74
Bartholin cyst, 68
Burn surface area, 72
Burns, 53, 71–74

## C
Cellulitis, 7, 8, 57, 58, 61, 65, 68–70, 76, 77
Chronic wound, 10, 59, 75–79
Contaminated wound, 19, 23, 33

## D
Debridement, 7, 14, 15, 25, 76
Decubitus ulcer, 79–81
   staging classifications, 78
Diabetes, 7, 9–11, 61, 75, 77

## E
Edema, 10, 57–60, 75–78

## F
Fever, 58, 62, 66, 67
Fibrosis, 3, 19, 21
Foreign body, 17, 66
Fracture, 14, 43

## H
Hemorrhage, 29, 30, 57
Hemostasis, 2, 13–15, 20, 30, 60
Hidradenitis suppurativa (HS), 67, 69–70
Horizontal mattress sutures, 42, 44, 46–48, 52

## I
Inflammation, 1, 2, 7, 8, 17, 21, 22, 33, 48, 59,
     61, 62, 65, 67–70
Irrigation, 7, 14, 16, 65, 66, 76

## N
Necrotizing fasciitis, 66
Nonabsorbable suture, 22

## P
Paronychia, 61, 64–65
Pilonidal cyst, 67–68

© Springer International Publishing Switzerland 2016
B. Busse, *Wound Management in Urgent Care*,
DOI 10.1007/978-3-319-27428-7